CANCER
The Misguided Cell

David M. Prescott
UNIVERSITY OF COLORADO

Abraham S. Flexer

SINAUER ASSOCIATES INC. • PUBLISHERS
Sunderland, Massachusetts

TO OUR PARENTS

CANCER: THE MISGUIDED CELL

Copyright © 1982 by David M. Prescott and Abraham S. Flexer. All rights reserved. This book may not be reproduced in whole or in part for any purpose whatsoever, without permission from the publisher. For information address Sinauer Associates, Inc., Publishers, Sunderland, Massachusetts 01375.

Printed in U.S.A.

Library of Congress Cataloging in Publication Data
Prescott, David M., 1926–
Cancer: the misguided cell.
Includes bibliographical references and index.
1. Cancer.   2. Oncology—Popular works. I. Flexer, Abraham S.   II. Title.   [DNLM: 1. Cells.   2. Neoplasms.   QZ 200 P929c]
RC263.P728   1981   616.99'4071   81-9033
ISBN 0-87893-707-2   AACR2

9 8 7 6 5 4 3 2

Contents

Preface

Cancer has touched our families and will likely touch yours, as well. This disease now strikes about one American in four, and kills about one in five. Yet there are few sources of information about the biology of cancer that are both reliable and accessible to undergraduates as well as to interested laypersons. This book is intended to be such a resource, with central ideas about the nature of cancer presented as far as possible in clear, generally nontechnical terms.

We have tried to write a book that will serve the reader both now and in the future. We offer an overview of what recent research has revealed about the causes of cancer, about how it can be treated and might be prevented. This overview is developed on a foundation of knowledge gained from basic research into the behavior and activities of cells, both normal and cancerous. Such knowledge is likely to endure longer than particular details about this cancer or that cancer-causing agent, this or that treatment. It is this basic knowledge that will help the interested reader to become informed about cancer and to remain informed; to sort out conflicting claims and counter-claims about alleged causes and cures that will continue to appear in the popular media.

Two themes dominate this book. One is that cancers begin when individual cells of the body suffer particular kinds of genetic changes, called mutations. These cancer-causing genetic changes result in the loss of normal controls over key cellular processes, converting a normal cell into one whose descendants may become a cancer. An overwhelming body of observations, experiences, and experiments support this mutational view. It has become a powerful principle around which to organize nearly all of what is known about the causes and nature of cancer, and so we use this principle as a major theme.

Cancer can be regarded, at least in part, as a social disease brought on by environmental pollution and by life-styles that involve potentially avoidable contacts with cancer-causing agents. This is the book's second major theme: that preventing cancer is a more effective approach than permitting it to develop, then trying to cure it. One third of the book is devoted to documenting what is known about the various agents—chemicals, radiation, and viruses—that are implicated in causing the kinds of genetic changes that result in cancers. This knowledge provides each person with a scientific basis for personal choices that minimize one's own exposure to cancer-causing agents; and it provides each citizen with a rational basis for evaluating social policies that affect the recognition and dissemination of known or potential cancer-causing agents. Prudent personal and social actions, we argue, offer the best long-range strategy for reducing cancer's now horrifying toll.

In developing these and other themes, we have tried to avoid both needless complexity and the complementary hazard of lapsing into misleading oversimplification. Nevertheless, some of the explanations remain more complex than we would wish. One reason for this is that some aspects of cancer are inherently technical. Another reason is more basic and unavoidable. Many questions about the nature of cancer simply cannot now be answered, and grappling with an incomplete account is always more difficult than presenting a comprehensive one. It is our conviction that the information included in this book will turn out to be a set of enduring insights into the nature of cancer. Knowledge is power, and knowledge of cancer—even incomplete knowledge—is a step toward developing the power to reduce cancer's devastation.

Many people contributed generously to this book. Our families have helped most, especially Gayle E. Prescott, who typed more drafts of the manuscript than any of us cares to recall. Particular thanks for contributing Chapter 12 (which discusses important psychosocial aspects of cancer) go to Dr.

Laurie Engelberg of the Department of Sociology, California State University at Fullerton, and to Mr. Lee H. Hilborne, University of California at San Diego. Dr. Engelberg teaches a course on the social aspects of cancer, and Mr. Hilborne is Chair of the Biology of Cancer Subcommittee of the California Division of the American Cancer Society. Both are also members of the Public Education Committee of the California Division of the American Cancer Society. Careful reviews of the manuscript and many helpful suggestions were offered by Prof. Michael B. Shimkin, Department of Community Medicine, University of California at San Diego School of Medicine, and by Prof. Albey M. Reiner, Department of Microbiology, University of Massachusetts. We did not, of course, accept all the advice offered us, and so whatever flaws exist are ours alone. D. M. Prescott expresses his appreciation to the Alexander von Humboldt Foundation, Federal Republic of Germany, for providing the opportunity to work on this book with the award of a U.S. Senior Scientist Prize. D. M. Prescott prepared much of the manuscript while a guest in the Genetics Institute, Justus Liebig University, Giessen, West Germany; he expresses his great appreciation to Professor F. Anders for his generous hospitality.

We sincerely hope that the reader finds this book informative and helpful, both in understanding cancer and in acting to prevent it.

DAVID M. PRESCOTT
ABRAHAM S. FLEXER

—————————I—————————

The Dimensions
of Cancer

C ANCER is an ancient disease. It has afflicted our ancestors throughout human history and almost certainly throughout human evolution. Egyptian medical tracts 3500 years old describe diseases today recognizable as cancer.[1,*] More direct evidence of cancer's antiquity is seen in distinctively scarred mummies and skeletons of ancient cancer victims (Figure 1).

Cancer has always been a much-feared although, until recently, a seldom-encountered scourge. But within the last century or so, the situation has changed dramatically. Cancer now ranks second only to heart disease as a major cause of death in the United States and is similarly devastating in the rest of the world. During 1981, in the United States alone, more than 800,000 people will develop cancer and about 420,000 people will die of cancer. Put in another way, at least one of every four Americans alive today will develop at least one cancer; one of every five Americans alive today will be killed by cancer. Reasons for this substantial rise in the incidence of cancer in modern times are now understood at least in general terms, and these reasons form one of the main themes of this book.

* These superscript numbers refer to comments and bibliographic notes which begin on page 279.

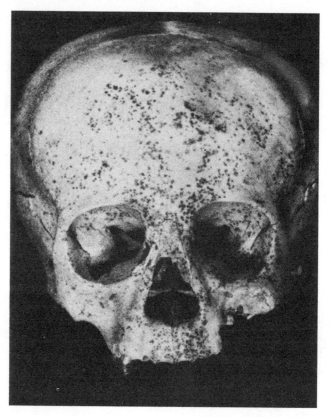

FIGURE 1   Skull of pre-Columbian Inca Indian afflicted with cancer many centuries ago. The small dark spots are scars left by a form of skin cancer that begins at a single site and spreads through the body.[2]

Infectious Diseases Gave Way to Degenerative Diseases

In 1850, about 1 of every 190 deaths in the United States was reported to be the result of cancer.[3] Cancer now accounts for one of every five deaths, and most of this increase occurred in this century (Figure 2). Ironically, these increases in cancer parallel social and economic improvements and have occurred despite advances in scientific knowledge and in medical practice.

Much of the increase in mortality from cancer and other

degenerative diseases is a result of decreases in mortality from infectious diseases. A century ago, infectious diseases were the major causes of deaths in the United States: tuberculosis, influenza, pneumonia, gastrointestinal infections, and diphtheria were all common and usually fatal. By the turn of the century, improvements in general nutrition, housing, public sanitation, and personal hygiene were reducing this toll. Even so, more than half of all deaths in the United States during 1900 were caused by infectious diseases (Figure 3).

During the first half of the twentieth century, general acceptance of the germ theory of disease led to a series of medical and public health advances that began to reduce both the frequency and the severity of infectious diseases. These included filtering and chlorinating municipal water supplies, improving the removal and treatment of sewage and other urban wastes, pasteurizing commercial dairy products, adopting antiseptic practices in hospitals and homes, improving methods of preserving and storing foods, administering specific vaccines and antitoxins to much of the population, and, most recently, de-

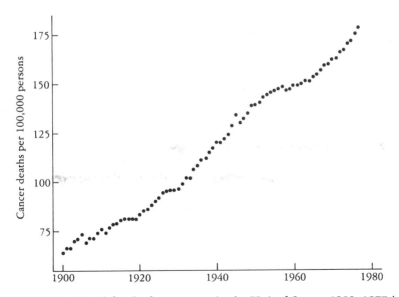

FIGURE 2   Total deaths from cancer in the United States, 1900–1977.[4]

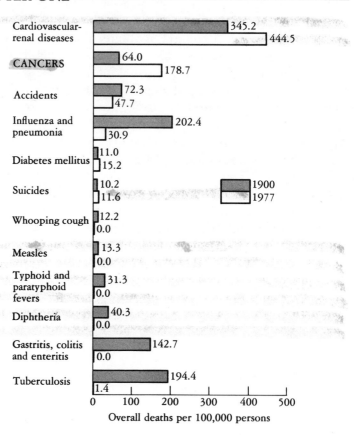

FIGURE 3 Overall deaths from various causes, United States, 1900 versus 1977.[4]

veloping highly effective antibiotics. These and other medical innovations have reduced current mortality from infectious diseases to about 1 death in 20 in the United States and in most developed countries. Principal beneficiaries of this defeat of infectious diseases have been those who were historically most vulnerable: the very young and the aged of both sexes and females in their adolescent and reproductive years.

Eliminating infectious diseases as major causes of death affected American society in many ways, not all of them anticipated. One predictable, salient effect was a sharp increase in the average life span. A white infant born at the turn of the century in the United States could expect to live fewer than 50 years (Figure 4) and was most likely to die of a cardiovascular–renal disease or of penumonia, tuberculosis, or another infectious disease. By 1975, life expectancy at birth increased

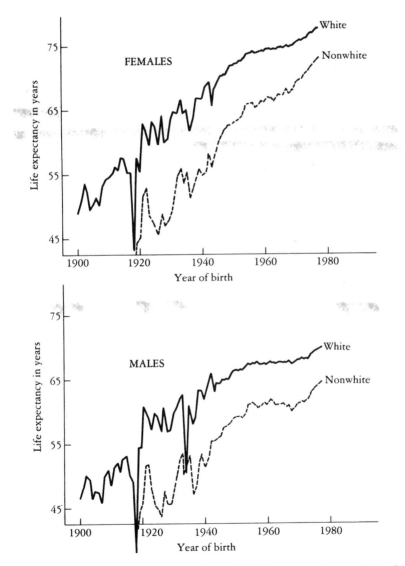

FIGURE 4 **Average life expectancies at birth by sex and race, United States, 1900–1977.**[4]

to more than 70 years for whites, and the most likely causes of death were cardiovascular diseases and cancer. Infectious diseases gave way to degenerative diseases as major causes of death (Table 1).

As life spans lengthened, the age structure of the United States population changed significantly. In 1900, only 4 percent of the population was 65 years old or older. By 1970, nearly 11 percent of the population was 65 or older (Figure 5). Figure 6 reveals why these changes in population structure are relevant to a discussion of mortality from cancer. Death from cancer is relatively uncommon among children and teenagers. For example, fewer than 6 persons per 100,000 at ages younger than 20 years die of cancer annually. At age 20 and beyond, the death rate from cancer accelerates rapidly, reaching annual rates

TABLE 1. The 15 major causes of death in the United States in 1977.[5]

Cause of Death	Number of Deaths	Percentage of Total Deaths	
1. Heart diseases	718,850	37.8	⎫ 58.2
2. Cancer	386,686	20.4	⎭
3. Cerebrovascular disease	181,934	9.6	
4. Accidents	103,202	5.4	
5. Pneumonia and influenza	51,193	2.7	
6. Diabetes mellitus	32,989	1.7	
7. Cirrhosis of liver	30,848	1.6	
8. Arteriosclerosis	28,754	1.5	
9. Suicide	28,681	1.5	
10. Diseases of infancy	23,401	1.2	
11. Homicide	19,968	1.1	
12. Emphysema	16,376	0.9	
13. Congenital abnormalities	12,983	0.7	
14. Kidney diseases	8,519	0.5	
15. Septicemia and pyemia	7,112	0.4	
Other	248,101	13.0	
TOTAL	1,899,597	100	

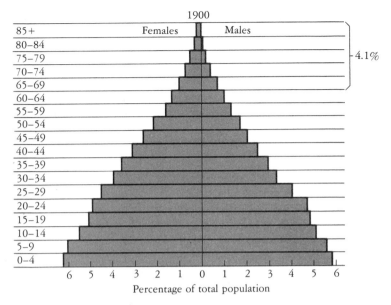

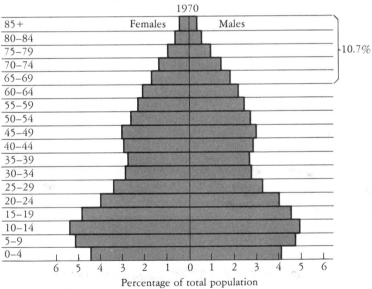

FIGURE 5 Age structures of the United States populations of 1900 and 1970 compared. These "population pyramids" show what part of the population belonged to each age group at each time. Each pyramid represents 100 percent of each population. The width of each bar to the right of the 0%-line represents the percentage of females of each age in the population. Males are represented to the left of the 0%-line.[6]

7

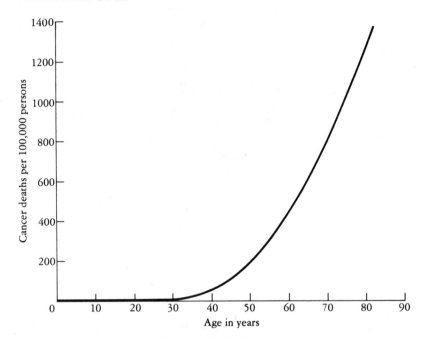

FIGURE 6 Number of persons per 100,000 of each age who died of cancer in the United States during 1979.[7]

of over 190 per 100,000 by age 50 and nearly 1300 per 100,000 by age 80. Overall this represents more than a 200-fold difference between rates among the very young and the very old. In short, as the life expectancy and average age of the United States population went up (Figure 4), so did the death rate from cancer (Figure 2). The obvious connection is the pattern of age-specific death rates from cancer shown in Figure 6. But what are the reasons for that pattern?

As discussed later in this chapter and more extensively in Chapter 6, most cancer (possibly more than 90 percent) results from cancer-causing agents in the environment. These carcinogens, particularly chemicals of various kinds, are in the foods we eat, in the air we breathe, in the water we drink, in the clothing we wear, sometimes in medicines we take, and in the workplaces where we earn our livings. The amounts and variety of these environmental carcinogens have increased sharply in the last half century and particularly in the last 25 years;[8] and they continue to increase rapidly.

The increase of the incidence of cancer with age and the induction of cancer by environmental agents are related in two ways. First, the longer an individual lives, the more likely it is that he or she will accumulate enough exposure to environmental carcinogens to develop cancer. Second, for almost all agents known to cause cancer, a delay of from 5 to 30 or more years separates the first exposure to a particular carcinogen and the detection of a cancer (Chapters 6 and 7). Thus, many years of chronic exposure to carcinogens usually precede the disease, a circumstance that displaces cancer into the older age groups.

Although half of the people who die of cancer today are over 65, the young are by no means spared. Cancer is now the most common cause of death *by disease* among children, ranking second only to accidents as a killer of children 14 years and younger (Table 2). Leukemia, cancer of the nervous system, and cancer of the lymphatic system now are the most common childhood cancers. This contrasts sharply with the situation in 1938, when cancer ranked *tenth* as a killer of children.[9] This shift did not result from a large absolute increase in childhood cancers but rather from the reduction of infectious diseases of childhood, as discussed earlier.

In any case, cancer now ranks as the second major cause of death in the United States: in 1977, heart diseases accounted for nearly 38 percent of all deaths and cancer for just over 20 percent (Table 1). The death rate for heart disease, however, has been declining slightly but significantly during the last several years, while the death rate for cancer has been increasing.[10]

This increase in overall cancer mortality in the United States and other developed countries is a particularly disturbing aspect of the cancer problem. From 1968 to 1977 (the last year for which complete data are available), the total annual cancer death rate in the United States increased from 159.4 to 178.7 per 100,000 people (Figure 2)—an increase in rate of over 12 percent in 9 years. Most of this increase was a result of the aging of the United States population, mentioned earlier (Figure 5). After correcting for this aging, the rate still increased

TABLE 2. Primary causes of death in children between ages 1 and 14 in the United States, 1977.[5]

Cause of Death	Annual Deaths	Percentage of Deaths
1. Accidents	9,502	45.5
2. Cancer	2,364	11.3
3. Congenital abnormalities	1,470	7.0
4. Homicide	766	3.7
5. Pneumonia and influenza	718	3.4
6. Heart diseases	540	2.6
7. Meningitis	454	2.2
8. Cerebrovascular diseases	274	1.3
9. Cystic fibrosis	249	1.2
10. Cerebral palsy	239	1.1
11. Suicide	190	0.9
12. Anemias	149	0.7
13. Bronchitis	126	0.6
14. Benign neoplasms	124	0.6
All other	3,721	17.8
TOTAL	20,866	99.9

a little more than 2.0 percent for the 9-year period.[11] Most (1.8 percent) of this age-adjusted increase took place in the final 4 years of the period (1973–1977), which suggests that the absolute rate of cancer death is beginning to climb more rapidly. A rate of increase of 1.8 percent in 4 years may sound modest, but if it were sustained to the year 2000, it would result in an additional 100,000 cancer deaths annually over the 1981 annual rate of approximately 420,000 cancer deaths. Most disturbing is the fact that the increase in the cancer death rate has and is taking place despite major efforts to improve and refine available proved methods for treating cancers and to introduce new techniques through research (see Chapter 10).

Cancers Vary in Frequency and Lethality

Changes in the overall rate of cancer mortality reflect changes in mortality rates for each individual kind of cancer. Figure 7 shows changes from 1930 to 1976 in the United States for

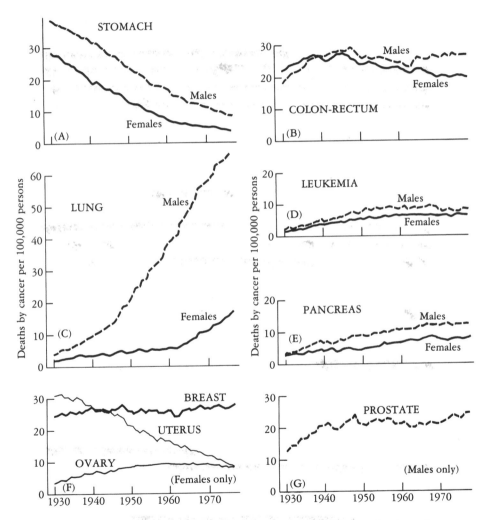

FIGURE 7 Age-adjusted cancer death rates for cancers of selected sites in United States population, 1930–1976.[12]

several major kinds of cancers in each sex. There is a striking decrease in mortality from stomach cancer in both men and women (Figure 7A): it was the most common form of cancer in 1930 but is now only the fourth (in women) or fifth (in men) most common. This decrease in mortality from stomach cancer comes almost entirely from a true decrease in the frequency of the disease in the United States and not from better treatment.[12] The reason for this dramatic decrease is not known, but the decrease may be related to changes in the American diet, for example, the year-round intake of vitamin C in fresh and frozen fruits and vegetables. Vitamin C is an antioxidant that may be important in preventing the formation in the stomach of carcinogenic chemicals from certain foods. In any event, the decrease in deaths caused by stomach cancer provides an important clue about cancer prevention. Unfortunately, we have not yet been able to exploit or even to understand this lead.

Mortality from cancer of the uterine cervix has also declined sharply (Figure 7F). In this case, the decrease reflects earlier diagnosis and improved treatment as well as decreased frequency of the disease.[13] Deaths from cancer of the rectum and colon (Figure 7B) have also declined slightly in females (with no decline in males), primarily because of a decrease in new cases of the disease. This decline is also presumably related to diet, but the connection is still unknown and is puzzling in view of the sex-related difference.[12]

The most striking increase shown in Figure 7 is that for lung cancer deaths in both sexes. In 1930, lung cancer killed 3 out of every 100,000 men each year and fewer women. At that time, lung cancer ranked eighth in the United States as a cause of cancer deaths in both sexes. By 1970 lung cancer killed 47 out of every 100,000 men annually, and by 1976 the annual toll reached 54 per 100,000. Lung cancer now ranks *first* among causes of cancer deaths in men. Mortality from this disease continues to rise faster than for any other cause of death, cancer or otherwise. The rise is primarily, but not exclusively, a result of exposure to tobacco smoke (see Chapter 7).

Among women lung cancer increased slowly but steadily

from 1930 to 1960, at which time deaths from this disease began to accelerate more rapidly. Deaths from lung cancer among women increased about 9-fold from 1930 to 1976 and continue to rise sharply.[12] If the present course of increase is sustained until the mid 1980s, more women will die of lung cancer than of breast cancer.[14] That would make lung cancer *the* leading cause of cancer deaths among women. The overall increase in lung cancer deaths exceeds by a substantial margin what little progress has been made in reducing deaths from other cancers.

Figure 8 summarizes for each sex the frequency of and mortality from cancers of major organs. The differences are substantial and not fully understood. It is clear that the high rates of lung cancer are a consequence of inhaling carcinogens in tobacco smoke and other air pollutants, such as asbestos (Chapter 7). Reasons for other differences among organs and between the sexes are less clear. Some of these differences, when explained, may yield important clues about the nature of cancer and of carcinogenesis. Time and future research will tell.

The economic costs of cancer are also depressing. Earnings lost by United States cancer victims during their illnesses and by premature death were estimated at about $15 billion during 1975. Additionally, direct costs of treating these victims was over $5 billion.[15] These direct costs of over $20 billion a year pale into insignificance when compared with the pain and suffering that the disease inflicts (see Chapter 12).

Most Cancers Are Caused by Environmental Factors

In principle there are two ways in which cancer might arise. First, a cancer might result from some error in a cellular process, for example, during the duplication of the genes when a cell reproduces (Chapter 3). Such errors might occasionally occur "spontaneously," that is, independently of external agents, and might be an intrinsic basis for cancer. Although certainly possible, intrinsic causes are not likely to account for more than a tiny fraction of human cancer. In any case, it is very unlikely that we could ever devise ways to prevent such

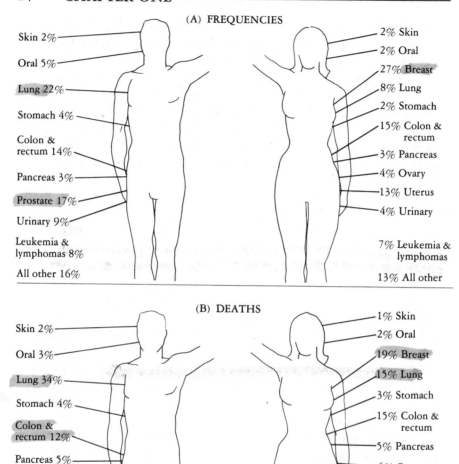

(A) FREQUENCIES

Skin 2%
Oral 5%
Lung 22%
Stomach 4%
Colon & rectum 14%
Pancreas 3%
Prostate 17%
Urinary 9%
Leukemia & lymphomas 8%
All other 16%

2% Skin
2% Oral
27% Breast
8% Lung
2% Stomach
15% Colon & rectum
3% Pancreas
4% Ovary
13% Uterus
4% Urinary
7% Leukemia & lymphomas
13% All other

(B) DEATHS

Skin 2%
Oral 3%
Lung 34%
Stomach 4%
Colon & rectum 12%
Pancreas 5%
Prostate 10%
Urinary 5%
Leukemia & lymphomas 9%
All other 16%

1% Skin
2% Oral
19% Breast
15% Lung
3% Stomach
15% Colon & rectum
5% Pancreas
6% Ovary
5% Uterus
3% Urinary
9% Leukemia & lymphomas
17% All other

FIGURE 8 Cancers and cancer deaths by sex and site, estimated for the United States, 1981. (A) Relative frequencies of various kinds of cancers. (B) Relative frequencies of deaths caused by various kinds of cancers. Because they are so easily cured, carcinoma *in situ* of the uterine cervix (over 45,000 new cases annually) and non-melanoma skin cancer (about 400,000 new cases annually) are excluded from these data.[12]

intrinsic cancers. Second, cancer might result from external agents that enter and affect cells, thereby triggering cancers. Environmental agents such as radiation, chemical carcinogens, and possibly viruses are known or suspected to cause many (probably most) human cancers.

We know, for example, that before adequate precautions were adopted, radiologists and X-ray technicians had much higher rates of cancer than other physicians and medical technicians. Infants treated with X rays to reduce enlarged thymus glands sustain an 83-fold greater rate of thyroid cancer later in life.[16] Excessive exposure to X rays can cause cancer in virtually any tissue.

Many radioactive substances are potent carcinogens. The survivors of the atomic bombs in Hiroshima and Nagasaki, uranium miners, and others occupationally exposed to radioactive substances all have significantly higher rates of cancer (especially leukemia and thyroid cancers) than the general population. Chronic, excessive exposure to the ultraviolet rays in sunlight is responsible for most skin cancers. These and other links between radiation and cancer are examined in Chapter 8.

Carcinogenic chemicals, because they are so widespread in our environment and because exposure to them is often massive and prolonged, are responsible for more cancer than radiation. The most notorious example, of course, is tobacco smoke, the chemical carcinogens of which now account for between one-fourth and one-third of *all* cancer deaths in the United States, that is, between 95,000 and 125,000 deaths per year.[17] Other chemical carcinogens, such as vinyl chloride, asbestos, and various organic and some inorganic chemicals cause excess cancers among industrial workers and, in some instances, in their families (Chapter 7). People who live in large cities, almost all of which have polluted air, develop cancers of the trachea, bronchi, lungs, and colon at higher rates than people who live in rural areas.[18] Similar cancers are also associated with the paper, chemical, and petroleum industries. This connection is exemplified by the high rates of tracheal, bronchial, and lung cancer along the United States Gulf Coast (Figure 9).

The importance of viruses in human cancer is much less certain. Epstein-Barr virus causes infectious mononucleosis and

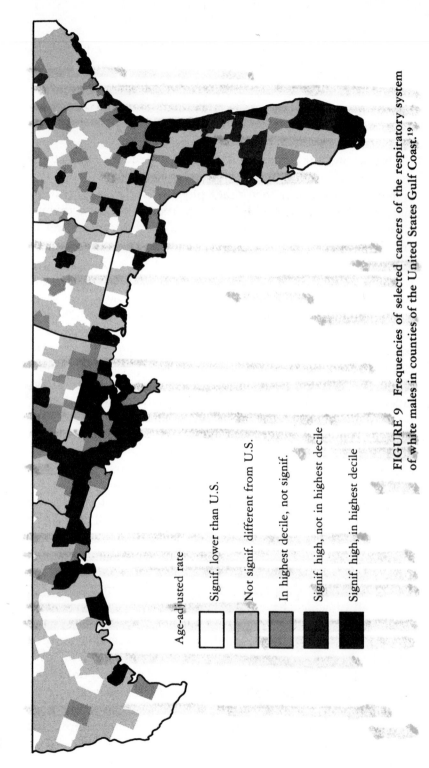

Age-adjusted rate

☐ Signif. lower than U.S.

☐ Not signif. different from U.S.

☐ In highest decile, not signif.

☐ Signif. high, not in highest decile

■ Signif. high, in highest decile

FIGURE 9 Frequencies of selected cancers of the respiratory system of white males in counties of the United States Gulf Coast.[19]

is related to the herpesviruses that cause cold sores and cankers. As described in Chapter 9, Epstein-Barr virus is consistently associated with Burkitt's lymphoma, which is a major form of cancer in Africa, and with nasal cancer in China. This association suggests but does not prove that viruses may account for some human cancers.

These are just a few examples of environmentally caused cancer, a topic to be covered in more detail in Chapters 6 through 9. The crucial questions considered here are how much of human cancer *is* caused by environmental agents and what are these agents? Identifying environmental causes of cancer is, of course, a precondition to eliminating them from the environment or at least for enabling an individual to minimize his or her personal risk of such exposure (see Chapter 11). It will probably be impossible to eliminate all environmental causes of cancer, even after all have been identified. For example, ionizing radiations from outer space cannot be eliminated and can be completely avoided only by living several miles underground. Cosmic radiation, however, accounts for no more than a tiny fraction of human cancer. Many of the other environmental agents responsible for the great bulk of human cancer could be eliminated or avoided by a combination of governmental and individual actions. What these are, and what progress is being made, are discussed in Chapter 11.

How much human cancer is, or might be, caused by environmental factors? One relatively simple approach to an answer to this question is to observe the rates of particular kinds of cancer in many places throughout the world. Assume that, for any particular kind of cancer, the lowest rate found in the world is the minimum possible rate—an irreducible background rate. Higher rates are then, at least presumptively, environmentally caused. For example, stomach cancer is 25 times more common in Japan than in Uganda (Table 3). Thus it could be inferred that the rate of stomach cancer in Japan could be reduced 25-fold (i.e., by 96 percent) if the causal factor(s) present in the Japanese environment but absent in the Ugandan environment were identified and could be removed from the Japanese environment.[21] Indeed, the rate of stomach cancer in Japan has been dropping for the last 25 years. During that same period, Japanese consumption of milk, eggs, meat, oil, and fruit has increased steadily, while the consumption of potatoes has fallen.[22] Which, if any, of these dietary or other changes is related to the observed decrease in stomach cancer is still unknown.

Mortality from stomach cancer in the United States has

TABLE 3. Range in rates of incidence of some common cancers.[20]

Type of Cancer	Area of High Incidence	Area of Low Incidence	Ratio of Rates	Percentage Environmental[a]
Esophagus	Iran	Nigeria	300-fold	99.7
Penis	Uganda	Israel	300-fold	99.7
Skin	Australia, Queensland	India, Bombay	200-fold	99.5
Liver	Mozambique	Norway	70-fold	98.6
Nasopharynx	Singapore (Chinese population)	England	40-fold	97.5
Bronchus	England	Nigeria	35-fold	97.1
Prostate	U.S.A. (Black population)	Japan	30-fold	96.7
Stomach	Japan	Uganda	25-fold	96.0
Mouth	India	Denmark	25-fold	96.0
Rectum	Denmark	Nigeria	20-fold	95.0
Uterine cervix	Colombia	Israel	15-fold	93.3
Colon	U.S.A., Connecticut[b]	Nigeria	10-fold	90.0
Uterus	U.S.A., Connecticut	Japan	10-fold	90.0
Ovary	Denmark	Japan	8-fold	87.5
Breast	U.S.A., Connecticut	Uganda	5-fold	80.0
Pancreas	New Zealand (Maori population)	Uganda	5-fold	80.0
Bladder	U.S.A., Connecticut	Japan	4-fold	75.0

[a]In region of highest incidence; calculated as 1 − (1/ratio of rates).
[b]Connecticut is cited in this table because the Connecticut Cancer Registry has kept careful records for many years.

dropped almost 4-fold since 1930 (Figure 7A), also presumably because of changes in diet. Such unexplained decreases within a population rule out genetic differences in predisposition to particular cancers among different nationalities and ethnic groups. Thus it might be argued that the 4-fold higher rate of stomach cancer in Japan compared to the United States[22] was due to genetic factors that make Japanese more susceptible to stomach cancer. The continuing 25-year-long decrease in stomach cancer in Japan, however, rules against such an explanation. In addition, Japanese who migrate to the United States acquire the lower United States rate of stomach cancer within one to two generations.[23] Most stomach cancer in Japan, possibly 96 percent or more as indicated by the Ugandan rate, is environmentally caused and therefore potentially preventable.

Other comparisons from Table 3 can be cited. The incidence of esophageal cancer is 300 times higher in Iran than in Nigeria, which suggests that 99.7 percent of all esophageal cancer in Iran may be environmentally caused and thus preventable, at least in principle.[24] Prostate cancer is 30 times more common among blacks in the United States than among Japanese in the United States, and nasopharyngeal cancer is 40 times more common among the Chinese of Singapore than among the English of Singapore. These latter figures imply that 96.7 and 97.5 percent of these cancers, respectively, may be preventable. Finally, it is again worth citing tobacco smoke as an environmental cause of cancer. From 1930 to 1978, the rate of lung cancer among United States males increased 18-fold (Figure 7C), and even the 1930 rate was at least in part a result of smoking tobacco. From the strong correlation between smoking cigarettes and rates of lung and other cancers (Chapter 7), it may reasonably be estimated that perhaps up to one-third of *all* cancer deaths in men in the United States could be prevented by eliminating only *one* environmental carcinogen, tobacco smoke.[17]

Such data on changing rates of cancer within particular regions of the world and on differences in rates among regions suggest that 90 percent of all human cancer is potentially preventable.[25] Indeed, this estimate may be conservative, because

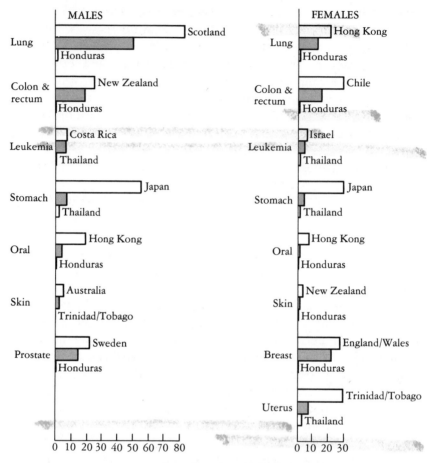

Age-adjusted cancer death rates
per 100,000, 1974–1975

FIGURE 10 Deaths from common cancers. The United States (gray bars) is compared with other countries with high death rates for these particular cancers. Bars show age-adjusted rates per 100,000 persons of each sex. Data are taken from a list of 46 countries with the highest and very low rates for each cancer.[12]

even the lowest observed rate for a given cancer might be substantially reduced if the causal agent(s) could be identified and removed from the local environment.

The magnitude of the opportunity for preventing cancer

deaths is suggested by Figure 10 and Table 4. Figure 10 compares the death rates from common cancers in the United
States with the corresponding rates in countries with the highest reported rates and particularly low (*not* the lowest known)
rates for those cancers. In each case, the death rate in the
United States is intermediate but significantly higher than the
lowest rate listed. Table 4 indicates that more than 170,000
cancer deaths might be avoided annually in the United States
alone if the death rates for these common cancers could be
reduced to those that prevail in countries with low (not the
lowest) rates.

Much work currently seeks to identify environmental carcinogens, particularly chemical carcinogens. A major part of this
work is epidemiological: the environments, living habits, and

TABLE 4. Cancer deaths in the United States, 1974–1975, that
might have been prevented if the United States death rate for
each type of cancer listed had been reduced to the lowest rate
shown in Figure 10. Because the lowest cancer death rates shown
in Figure 10 are not the lowest known, these figures may underestimate significantly the number of lives that might, in principle, have been saved.[26]

Type of Cancer	Potentially Preventable Deaths among:	
	Males	Females
Lung	52,004	12,034
Colon and rectum	19,722	16,300
Leukemia	6,228	3,938
Stomach	5,190	2,844
Oral	4,774	1,641
Skin	2,699	1,641
Prostate	14,947	—
Breast	—	23,959
Uterus	—	4,485
TOTALS	105,564 172,406	66,842

occupations of peoples throughout the world with particularly high or low rates of cancer are being scrutinized for clues to the origins of various kinds of cancers (Chapter 6). Enough has already been learned to enable the institution of some major preventative measures, although for cultural, political, and economic reasons, such steps toward protecting ourselves from cancer are agonizingly slow (Chapter 11).

A major, nonepidemiological approach to identifying cancer-causing agents is to test suspected carcinogens with laboratory animals. Unfortunately, testing a single suspected agent in animals may cost some $400,000 and takes several years. Newer tests for carcinogenicity that take a few days or weeks and cost far less are rapidly being refined.

Although such tests are already widely respected, they are not universally accepted for a variety of scientific and extrascientific reasons. Chapter 6 and later chapters will include a discussion of the rationale of these tests and what they can and cannot reveal.

Treatments for Major Cancers Are Not Very Effective

Some kinds of cancers can be treated successfully, others cannot. The differences reflect factors such as how early each kind of cancer can be detected, how often and how quickly the cancer spreads to other organs, how accessible the cancer is, and how amenable each is to treatment. The overall effectiveness of current treatments is suggested by Figure 11, which shows the 5-year survival, by sex, for the 25 most common cancers in the United States. At least 80 percent of persons with lip and thyroid cancer survive at least 5 years, but only 8 percent of men with lung cancer and 13 percent of women with lung cancer are alive 5 years after their disease is first diagnosed. The 5-year survival figures for esophageal, liver, and pancreatic cancers are still grimmer. Even for those cancers in which the 5-year survival rate is high, it must be remembered that 5-year survival does not necessarily represent a permanent cure; in many cases recurrences develop after 5 years.

FIGURE 11   Five-year survival rates by sex for major kinds of cancer ▶ in the United States population, 1965–1969.[12]

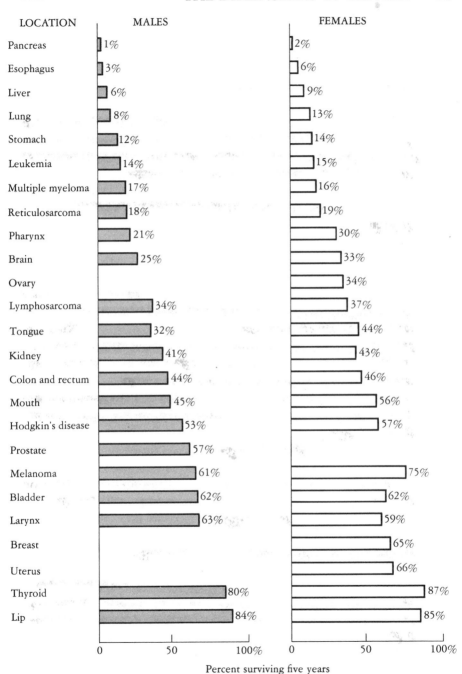

LOCATION	MALES	FEMALES
Pancreas	1%	2%
Esophagus	3%	6%
Liver	6%	9%
Lung	8%	13%
Stomach	12%	14%
Leukemia	14%	15%
Multiple myeloma	17%	16%
Reticulosarcoma	18%	19%
Pharynx	21%	30%
Brain	25%	33%
Ovary		34%
Lymphosarcoma	34%	37%
Tongue	32%	44%
Kidney	41%	43%
Colon and rectum	44%	46%
Mouth	45%	56%
Hodgkin's disease	53%	57%
Prostate	57%	
Melanoma	61%	75%
Bladder	62%	62%
Larynx	63%	59%
Breast		65%
Uterus		66%
Thyroid	80%	87%
Lip	84%	85%

Percent surviving five years

For these and other reasons, an overall cure rate for cancer is difficult to estimate. Because cancer tends to be a disease of older people (Figure 6), many cancer victims die of other causes (e.g., heart disease or pneumonia) before their cancer kills them. Thus the actual cure rate cannot be estimated simply by subtracting the total number of people who die of the disease from the total number who acquire it. Estimates of the actual cure rate range as high as 40 percent; the true value is probably somewhat less than 30 percent.[27] In any case, the majority of people who have cancer eventually die from it.

It will probably be necessary to accept the premise that there is some lower limit beyond which cancer cannot be prevented even if a society were sensible enough to exploit what has and is being learned about causes and prevention. Because the overall cure rate is probably close to 30 percent, it must also be admitted that current methods of treating people afflicted with the disease are not adequate. Each of the three major methods of treatment—surgery, radiation therapy, and chemotherapy—has limits, as discussed in Chapter 10. Surgery and radiation are not usually effective once a cancer has spread (metastasized) from its tissue of origin, and spreading is one of the principal attributes of malignant cancers (Chapter 2). Chemotherapy uses highly toxic chemicals that tend to kill at least some kinds of cancer cells more rapidly than they kill normal cells. Some advantage can be gained in treating some cancers by using combinations of two or more such drugs. But the advantage in chemotherapy often is not great, and the use of chemotherapeutic drugs other than hormones is limited by the severe side effects caused by damage to normal cells. For some cancers, the combination of two or more therapies (for example, surgery followed by radiotherapy or chemotherapy) is more effective than either treatment alone.

The effectiveness of a treatment for cancer should not be judged only in terms of cures. Some current treatments extend, often by many years, the life spans of cancer patients, often without reducing significantly the quality of the individual's life. These must be recognized as effective treatments, even if subsequent recurrences of the cancer are eventually fatal.

On balance, current treatments are not altogether effective, and although no one can predict what tomorrow's research may yield, prospects for fundamentally more effective treatments presently are dim. Prevention remains the more promising approach for the future—prevention based on an understanding of the nature and origin of cancer. This book offers to the interested nonspecialist an understanding of how cancer can be minimized by making prudent choices of behaviors that reduce the personal risk of developing the disease.

A central theme of this book is that cancer begins when individual cells lose control over their activities. The next two chapters explain how normal cells control their activites and how those controls can be disrupted in ways that lead to cancer. The vast majority of these disruptions result from changes to a cell's genetic program that ultimately directs normal controls. Thus, an understanding of genetics is central to an understanding of the origins of cancer (Chapter 4), as is an understanding of the basis for familial differences in susceptibility to cancer (Chapter 5). An introduction to the central ideas about cancer-causing agents (Chapter 6) leads to separate chapters about each of the three major classes of cancer-causing agents: chemicals, radiations, and viruses (Chapters 7, 8, and 9, respectively). Following a chapter on current and prospective treatments for cancer (Chapter 10), Chapter 11 outlines what each person can do to reduce his or her personal risk of cancer. A final chapter explores some of the psychological and social effects of cancer on its victims and their families and friends.

2

The Cellular Basis of Cancer

CANCER, like all organic diseases, results from the misfunctioning of one of the many cells that make up the body. Cancers generally begin when a single normal cell is converted into a cancer cell, a conversion that is not yet fully understood. Each descendant of the single cancer cell is also a cancer cell and all, in turn, produce more cancer cells. Whatever the nature of the conversion, then, it is transmitted from one cell generation to the next at each cell division.

The misfunctions characteristic of cancer cells are fundamentally different from the misfunctions that occur in other diseases. In almost all other diseases, the misfunction stems from the injury or death of normal cells. Bacteria that cause tuberculosis, for example, destroy lung cells, and bacteria that cause diphtheria produce a poison that kills cells of many tissues by blocking protein synthesis. Similarly, polio viruses destroy nerve cells, and hepatitis viruses destroy liver cells.

Cancer cells, by contrast, are not injured, nor are they dying, nor do they directly destroy other cells. They are, by most criteria, remarkably healthy. Cancer cells have two important properties that underlie the nature of the disease. First, cancer cells grow and divide with less restraint, whereas growth and division of normal cells are closely regulated. Second, cancer cells do not differentiate normally and therefore do not perform their normal functions in the body. In particular, cancer cells do not die on schedule. Eventually, the resulting overgrowth of misfunctioning cells interferes in some way with the activities of normal cells and tissues. The usual consequence of the unrestrained formation of cancer cells is the death of the person in whom the cancer formed.

Much Cancer Research Is at the Cellular or Molecular Level

A great deal remains to be learned about cancer but, as in all basic research, we have no certain way to estimate the magnitude or even the nature of things still undiscovered. Sustained research yields a stream of new observations, data, and interpretations, some of which will turn out to be more relevant to cancer than others. We can never be certain beforehand which new observation, which yet-to-be-discovered fact will be most useful. Such uncertainty about the unknown is one reason why, to those outside a field of research, and sometimes even to those in the field, the course of research may at times seem erratic, even disorganized. The difficulty of following a straight path to a goal of unknown dimensions and location is obvious. Progress is best achieved by a systematic closing-in on the target from many directions, using clues provided by many lines of research. Experience in other fields of science suggests that such a closing-in can be made systematic by adopting a few guiding principles of great generality and stability.

One such guiding principle, shared by many, perhaps most, members of today's research community is reflected in the opening paragraphs of this chapter. This principle is that an understanding of cancer can best be achieved through an understanding of controls over growth, reproduction, and specialization of normal cells and an understanding of how these controls fail in cancer cells. The sources of the deep commitment to this principle are numerous and complex and will become clear as you progress through this book. One such source is a century of great success in medical research and practice based on the principle that organic diseases are cellular phenomena. The defeat of the formerly devastating infectious diseases discussed in Chapter 1 stems largely from this cellular view. A second source of this cellular view derives from the continuing success of a particular approach to biological and medical research. It is that both the normal and the abnormal can most fruitfully be investigated through research programs that consistently compare each with the other rather than merely studying the abnormal by itself.

Accelerating progress in unraveling details of the structures and functions of normal and various kinds of abnormal cells has generated a sense of optimism that the cellular approach will eventually pay off. Progress during the last decade has been particularly rapid and the level of optimism has been correspondingly high. True, researchers in all periods fuel their efforts with such optimism; no one would pursue a problem if convinced of its ultimate unsolvability. Yet, with each passing year, the grounds for this optimism that the details of normal cellular activities and controls are ultimately knowable, perhaps even soon, have become progressively firmer.

The quest to understand normal and cancer cells has driven researchers to focus on progressively smaller dimensions: from organs and tissues to cells and from cells to subcellular organelles and to macromolecules. This progression of focus reflects another guiding principle—a relatively recent one—namely, to understand cancer we must ultimately seek explanations at the molecular level. Yet research at each level of organization has yielded some insights not accessible at any other level. Research at each level has also complemented and extended independent research at other levels. This chapter and Chapters 3 and 4 also follow this progression and focus on successively smaller dimensions.

The cellular and molecular views merge in a working hypothesis that dominates much thinking about cancer and much of this book. Put simply, the hypothesis is that cancers result from mutations in genes that normally control the reproduction and differentiation of cells. Thus, a major goal of current basic research on cancer has been to unravel at the molecular level the mechanisms by which normal cells control their growth, reproduction, and differentiation and to understand how these controls are different or defective in cells we recognize as cancerous. The balance of this chapter focuses largely on current views of such controls and their failure in cancer cells. We begin with the activities of cells in the healthy adult.

Turnover of Normal Cells Is Closely but Flexibly Regulated

Among the tissues of an average adult human are about 100 different types of cells that together add up to about 300 trillion (10^{14}) cells. Some types of cells (nerve cells, for example) live for many years; others (such as white blood cells) have life spans of only a few days. Consider an intermediate example: the death and replacement of red blood cells in a healthy person. The body of an average adult contains about 25 trillion red blood cells. An average red blood cell lives for about 120 days. Thus, on average, a healthy adult forms 25 trillion red blood cells every 120 days to replace the 25 trillion red blood cells that die in that time. This translates to about 2.5 million cell divisions every *second*.[1] Biologists speak of the death and replacement of cells as TURNOVER and say that red blood cells *turn over* at the rate of 2.5 million per second.

Other kinds of cells, such as white blood cells and cells that line the intestinal tract, have much shorter life spans and correspondingly higher turnover rates. A conservative estimate is that, overall, about 10 million cells normally die and are replaced each second of every day during the adult life of the average person. A healthy adult thus produces nearly one trillion (10^{12}) cells each day.

The 100 or so cell types can be grouped into two large classes on the basis of their capacity to reproduce. Some types of cells do not reproduce in the adult: nerve cells, cells of the voluntary muscles, and muscle cells of the heart. All other types of cells are able to reproduce in the adult: blood cells, skin cells, liver cells, and so on. Among cells of the second class, reproduction often is normally suspended but may be resumed under certain conditions. A good example is provided by cells called osteocytes, some of which are buried within the hard substance of bones and seldom reproduce. If a bone is broken, osteocytes in the immediate vicinity of the injury will begin to reproduce and participate in repairing the damaged bone. Once the repair is completed, the reproduction of these cells again is suspended. An osteocyte may remain quiescent within a bone for many years, but within a few hours after a nearby break, such a cell may again begin to grow and reproduce.

This second class of cells, which may suspend but never relinquish the capacity to reproduce, includes a wide variety of cell types. Rates of reproduction vary considerably from type to type and may be extremely slow in some cases. The cells of normal skin are constantly dying and sloughing off, a process that is particularly apparent on the scalp where the dead cells can detach in clumps known as dandruff. This loss of cells from the skin is compensated for by the essentially continuous reproduction of cells in an underlying layer. White blood cells and cells that line the intestinal tract live for several days or less and must also be constantly replaced. By contrast, the rate at which liver cells die and are replaced by reproduction is almost imperceptibly small, and the turnover rate in the kidney is so slow that special methods are required to detect it.

In all of these tissues in which turnover occurs, the rate of cell reproduction is closely regulated. We mentioned that in the average adult 2.5 million red blood cells wear out and are destroyed every second. Normally these lost cells are exactly replaced by the reproduction of appropriate cells in the bone marrow. The rate of cell reproduction can be increased enormously when a tissue is injured or when many cells are lost. For example, bleeding stimulates the rapid reproduction of blood-forming cells of the bone marrow. Injuries to the skin— sunburn, heat burns, cuts—greatly accelerate the rate of cell division in the deeper layers of the skin, a response that speeds the repair of the injured area. If one kidney is removed from an animal, cells in the remaining kidney reproduce more rapidly; the remaining kidney thus enlarges and is able to carry the load normally shared by two kidneys. In each case, the timing and rate at which new cells form is precisely coordinated with the rate at which cells die or are lost. It is generally true that in each normal adult tissue in which cell turnover occurs, the rate of reproduction is closely but flexibly regulated; moreover, the new cells differentiate normally and perform all of the functions of lost cells.

Development Involves Reproduction and Differentiation of Cells

Perhaps the most momentous event in the life of a human being is the first—the brief but complex process termed fertilization (Figure 1). Shortly after egg and sperm fuse, the chro-

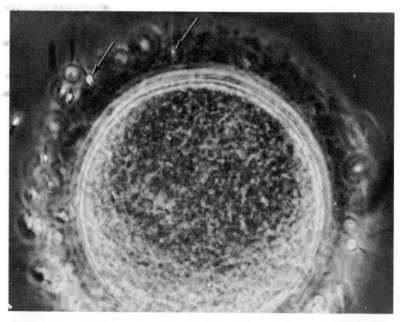

FIGURE 1 Fertilization of a human egg. Sperm cells (arrows) have become attached to the fuzzy material that encloses the egg. Many other sperm cells are visible here, but are out of focus. Once a single sperm enters the egg, the surface of the egg changes in a way that prevents penetration of any additional sperm.[2]

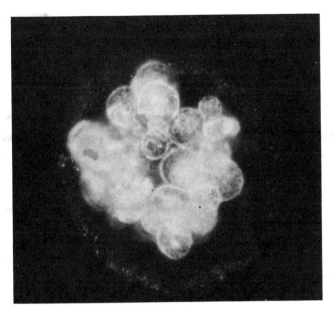

FIGURE 2   A human embryo in a very early stage of development. Following fertilization (Figure 1) the egg cell begins to divide. Within 5 or 6 days about 50 cells have been produced as shown here.[3]

mosomes of the sperm join the chromosomes in the egg to form a single, composite nucleus. About 24 hours after fertilization, the fertilized egg first divides. During the next several days, a series of cell divisions occurs at short intervals, resulting in a cluster of essentially identical cells (Figure 2).

From this point onward, continued rapid cell reproduction is accompanied by the specialization of various groups of cells for various tasks. The cells sort themselves first into layers, later into the organs and tissues that give the embryo and then the fetus their characteristic forms. This specialization of cells is collectively termed DIFFERENTIATION. The puzzle of differentiation lies in the facts that all the cells of the body carry the same genetic information, but that only part of the information is expressed in each differentiated cell. Somehow, as cells differentiate, each is channeled along one of many alternate paths so that different parts of the genetic information are expressed in different cell types, leading to different functions or behaviors. At birth, the human infant consists of about 5 trillion cells differentiated into the 100 or more different cell types mentioned earlier.

Throughout prenatal development and postnatal growth and development of the individual, the rates of cell reproduction and the processes of differentiation are precisely controlled. In certain instances, control means a complete repression of cell reproduction once the appropriate numbers and kinds are formed and become differentiated. This class of nondividing cell types, which includes nerve cells, cells of the voluntary muscles, and muscle cells of the heart, was mentioned earlier. Such cells cannot be replaced when lost through accident or disease. In other instances, cells continue to reproduce and differentiate at various rates through most of a person's life, for example, skin cells, cells of the blood-forming organs, and cells of the liver.

It is important to understand that the normal pattern of differentiation for a given cell type includes a programmed life span that often ends in the death of the fully differentiated cells. Several examples of such programmed cell death have already been mentioned, including red and white blood cells and the cells that line the digestive tract. Programmed cell death is also important during normal prenatal development. Fingers and toes, for example, form when blocks of cells in the early limb buds die on schedule.

Normal pre- and postnatal development and the continued well-being of the individual thus depend on the precise control of the turnover and differentiation of cells that retain the capacity to reproduce. So long as differentiated cells die on schedule and are replaced precisely (both in number and in kind), all is normal. Understanding the mechanisms by which these processes are precisely controlled in normal tissues is one of the major challenges in contemporary cell biology—and in cancer research.

Cancer Results from the Failure of Normal Controls

Disturbances in the normally precise control of the turnover and differentiation of cells may result in disease. If, for example, cell division throughout the body should cease altogether, the lining of the intestinal tract would disappear within a few days as the cells of that tissue completed their normal life spans. This would lead to uncontrollable diarrhea and, within a short time, to death by dehydration. By contrast, a disease known as polycythemia vera involves the uncontrolled overproduction of red blood cells. The circulatory system can become so clogged with the excess cells that it cannot function properly—with fatal results.

Cancer results from disruptions in the controls normally exerted over reproduction and differentiation. For example, certain white blood cells (called lymphocytes) ordinarily circulate in the body for a few days and then die. Dying is just as much a part of a normal program of differentiation as is acquiring the ability to engulf and destroy invading bacteria and viruses. In a healthy individual, lymphocytes are replaced by reproduction of special cells in the lymphatic system and in the bone marrow. These special cells form intermediate cells that differentiate into mature lymphocytes. In certain forms of leukemia, newly formed lymphocytes do not follow the normal developmental program: they do not differentiate fully, they do not acquire the capacity to destroy bacteria, and they do not die on schedule. Instead, these long-lived, defective cells persist in the circulatory system. As they accumulate and crowd out the normal cells of the blood, the body becomes progressively less able to defend itself against infections by bacteria, viruses, fungi, and other pathogenic agents. Understandably, the immediate cause of death associated with leukemia is sometimes a bacterial or viral infection.

The example of leukemia illustrates features common to all forms of cancer: the uncontrolled production of cells and the failure to differentiate normally. One key aspect of this abnormal differentiation is the greatly prolonged life spans of cancer cells compared with those of their normal counterparts; cancer cells are essentially immortal. Another aspect of abnormal differentiation is the failure of the cancer cells to develop the specialized functions of their normal counterparts. Therefore, much cancer research focuses on how reproduction and differentiation of normal cells are regulated, how the regulation fails in cancer cells, and how a normal cell is converted into a cancer cell.

The conversion of a normal cell to a cancer cell is, as mentioned earlier, a profound one: every descendant of the original cancer cell is also cancerous. A typical human cancer cell growing in artificial culture will, for example, divide about once every 24 hours.[4] At that rate, a single cancer cell would generate over one billion descendants in 30 days, a mass that would weigh about 1/60 of an ounce. In another 2 weeks, such a cancer would grow to over 17 trillion (10^{12}) cells, a mass of almost 20 pounds.[5] Fortunately, cancer cells do not reproduce nearly this rapidly in a body. A cancer cell normally requires months or years to give rise to a cancer mass of a few pounds. Thus, although cancer represents an overproduction of cells, cancer cells do not reproduce without restraint. In fact, some cancer cells may not even reproduce at particularly high rates. As we will discuss in Chapter 3, some types of normal cells (e.g., blood-forming cells and cells that line the intestine) reproduce much more rapidly than most kinds of cancer cells. But because cancer cells are immortal and misfunctional, they will, if unchecked by treatment, accumulate and fatally disrupt the body's functions. This may happen in a variety of ways, as described in the following section.

Cancers Usually Spread Throughout the Body

The first stage in the development of a cancer is, then, the transformation of a normal cell to a cell that reproduces and differentiates abnormally. The second stage is the spread of cancer cells to other organs of the body. Indeed, it is because cancer cells spread or METASTASIZE to other parts of the body that cancer is so difficult to deal with. Unfortunately, cancer is often first detected by symptoms of the secondary cancerous growths, called METASTASES, rather than by symptoms of the initial, primary cancer. Metastasis of cancer cells is the reason that early detection is essential (Chapter 10). If a cancer can be detected and removed before metastases occur, the chances for a cure are far better. Once cells detach from the primary cancer and begin to grow elsewhere in the body, the disease is much more difficult to treat; most individuals with metastases are eventually killed by the cancer.

Not all cells that become transformed lead to cancers. For reasons not yet understood, some cells in which differentiation and regulation of reproduction are defective do not metastasize. Rather, they form solid, well-defined tumors that remain surrounded by fibrous capsules. Some tumors of this type grow for a while and then spontaneously stop growing. Two quite common examples are FIBROMAS, which consist of masses of connective tissue and cells called fibroblasts, and LIPOMAS, which consist primarily of fat cells. Other noncancerous tumors may continue to grow and may reach enormous sizes. Growths that remain enclosed and do not spread, whether they stop growing or continue to enlarge, are called BENIGN tumors. They can almost always be completely cured merely by removing them surgically.

The way the word TUMOR is used sometimes creates confusion. Originally, the word meant any swelling. It has come to mean more specifically a swelling due to the abnormal growth of cells. If the mass of abnormal cells is encapsulated as just described, the growth is called a benign tumor. If the cells spread away from the initial, primary tumor, and metastasize to other parts of the body, the growth is said to be a MALIGNANT tumor. The word CANCER is generally used as a synonym for malignant tumor.

Technical names for tumors may also be confusing. In general, these names consist of a prefix that describes the tissue in which the tumor originates and a suffix that tells whether it is benign or malignant. Common prefixes include *fibro-* (fibrous or connective tissues), *adeno-* (glandular tissues), and *lipo-* (fat cells). Names for *benign* tumors are constructed from these prefixes and the suffix *-oma*—literally, a tumor. Thus FIBROMAS and ADENOMAS are benign tumors of connective and glandular tissues, respectively.

To distinguish *malignant* tumors, the roots *sarc-* (fleshy) and *carcino-* (crablike) are added. A FIBROSARCOMA is thus a malignant tumor of a connective tissue, and a LIPOSARCOMA, a malignant tumor of fat cells. These roots also reveal the embryonic origin of the tissue in question. Tissues derived from the middle of the three embryonic layers (mesoderm) give rise to sarcomas [for example, bone (osteosarcomas) and liposarcomas]. Tissues derived from the innermost and outermost embryonic layers (endoderm and ectoderm, respectively), give rise to carcinomas. For example, cancers of the liver are HEPATOCARCINOMAS, and cancers of pigment-forming skin cells are MELANOCARCINOMAS. These conventions are not universally followed, however; for example, hepatocarcinoma is usually contracted to HEPATOMA and melanocarcinoma to MELANOMA. Likewise, although leukemias and lymphomas are technically sarcomas, the former names are more commonly used.

Some cancers are more malignant than others. The degree of malignancy depends in part on the rate at which the cells reproduce, but a more critical property is how readily cells detach from the primary cancer and spread. Cancers that tend to metastasize quickly (i.e., when the number of cancer cells is still small) are generally more malignant. This is so because secondary cancers often form in tissues such as brain, lung, liver, or bones and are difficult to detect and usually difficult to treat. A secondary cancer may, in turn, metastasize and initiate tertiary cancers in still other locations. Skin cancers of the melanoma type are extremely malignant for just these reasons (Figure 1 in Chapter 1).

METASTASIS of cancer cells occurs in several steps. First, individual cells or loose clumps of cells may detach from the primary cancer. Cancer cells generally move actively, much as an ameba does. Although several kinds of normal cells, including white blood cells, are at least as motile as cancer cells, the normal counterparts of cancer cells generally are not. (Cells of benign tumors are usually enclosed by fibrous capsules and also tend to be much less motile, even when not enclosed.)

In addition to being motile, cancer cells generally do not adhere to one another or to normal cells. By contrast, normal cells of a given type, such as liver cells or kidney cells, usually adhere to one another to form well-defined tissues. There are exceptions to this generalization, of course, because some normal cells (white blood cells) move freely about the body. The important point is that cancer cells show less cell-to-cell adhesion than their normal counterparts, and this trait may be important in their ability to metastasize. This decreased cell-to-cell adhesion is accounted for by changes that occur in the surface of the cell membrane when a normal cell is converted to a cancer cell. The independent, wandering behaviors of cancer cells compared to their normal counterparts can be readily observed in artificial cultures.

Cancers Metastasize Through the Circulatory Systems

Metastasizing cancer cells may also penetrate the walls of blood vessels or lymphatic vessels (see later). Loosely clumped groups of cancer cells may be carried by the circulation to distant sites. There they may become lodged in narrow vessels or capillaries, invade other normal tissues, or invade one of the body's major cavities (e.g., the abdominal or chest cavities). As these metastases grow, they are penetrated by new blood vessels that then carry nutrients and oxygen to and wastes away from the secondary cancer. The blood- and lymph-circulating systems thus are important in the establishment and survival of metastases.

The heart pumps blood through a system of smaller and smaller arteries that branch to reach all parts of the body. From the smallest arteries, blood flows into a meshwork of fine capillaries. Blood in the capillaries releases nutrients and oxygen to the tissues and takes up carbon dioxide for transport to the lungs and waste products for transport to the kidneys. Blood then flows from the capillaries into a system of progressively larger veins that carry it back to the heart. Cancer cells may enter the blood by moving through the walls of capillaries in much the same way that normal white blood cells do (Figure 3). Once in the blood, cancer cells can be carried in a matter of minutes to any part of the body. Sarcomas in particular usually spread via the blood circulatory system.

Few people are familiar with the lymphatic system.[7] Although the blood circulatory system is two-way (delivering

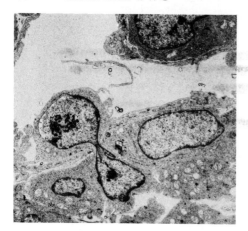
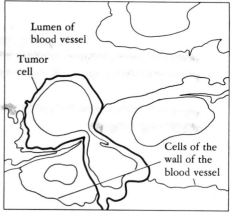

FIGURE 3   An electron micrograph showing a tumor cell in a rat squeezing through the wall of a small blood vessel to enter the circulatory system.[6]

blood to all the tissues of the body and returning it to the heart), the lymphatic system carries fluids in only one direction [from the tissues back toward the heart (Figure 4)]. The fluid carried in the lymphatic system is called LYMPH. It forms as blood serum filters across capillary walls into the tissues. An extensive system of lymphatic vessels collects lymph from all the tissues and empties it into the bloodstream just before the blood enters the heart. The lymphatic system thus collects but does not distribute lymphatic fluid.

At intervals along their routes, the lymphatic vessels lead into another component of the lymphatic system, the LYMPH NODES, which are enlargements in lymph vessels (Figure 4). Lymph filters through a lymph node and leaves by a continuation of the same lymphatic vessel that entered the node. Lymph nodes themselves are dense, compact collections of lymphocytes (white blood cells). Lymphocytes are added to the lymph fluid as it filters through successive lymph nodes, so that lymph is a thick, creamy-white fluid by the time it empties into a large vein near the heart. Recall that lymphocytes engulf invading bacteria; lymph nodes filter and destroy viruses and bacteria that may enter the lymphatic vessels from an infected tissue, blocking the spread of the infection.

Cancer cells, primarily carcinoma cells, may break away from a primary growth, move through a capillary wall, and enter a lymphatic vessel. Once in a lymphatic vessel, they may travel to any part of the body because the lymphatic system ultimately empties into the blood stream. However, lymph nodes along the drainage route may trap cancer cells and prevent their further spread. Because carcinomas so often spread by way of the lymphatic system, the lymph nodes on the drainage route away from a primary cancer are usually searched for

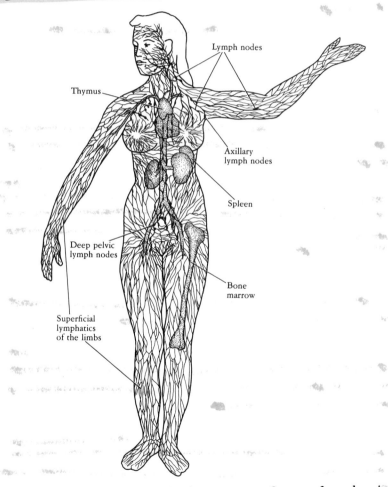

Lymph nodes

Thymus

Axillary lymph nodes

Spleen

Deep pelvic lymph nodes

Bone marrow

Superficial lymphatics of the limbs

FIGURE 4 The lymphatic circulatory system. See text for a description of the role of this system in the spread of cancer.

cancer cells when a cancer is removed by surgery. Finding cancer cells in a lymph node indicates that the cancer has already spread. Although lymph nodes may temporarily restrict the spread of cancer through the lymphatic route, eventually cancer cells escape from lymph nodes and metastasize throughout the body.

Lymph nodes usually occur in loose clusters; within a cluster, the more nodes that contain metastasizing cancer cells, the more advanced the spread of cancer and the poorer the prognosis. For example, the primary lymphatic drainage from each breast is toward the lymph nodes of the armpit. These lymph nodes are always examined when a breast with a cancer is removed during a mastectomy. If no lymph node contains cancer cells, the chances are good that the cancer had not spread and that the surgeon had removed all of the cancer. The more lymph nodes that contain cancer cells, the poorer the chance of a cure. The further course of the disease can be estimated from the number of lymph nodes that contain cancer cells. However, not detecting cancer cells in an adjacent lymph node does not guarantee absence of metastases. About 25 percent of women with cancer-negative lymph nodes in the armpit eventually develop metastases despite the surgery. Cancer cells that give rise to these metastases may have traveled a different route, for example, through lymph nodes below the breast bone. Cancer cells in these nodes are not ordinarily detected because the nodes are difficult to reach.

Cells probably break away continuously from primary cancers and enter lymphatic and blood vessels. In mice, breast cancers that have grown to about one-tenth of an ounce (about 3 grams) release several million cells a day into the blood. Few of the cancer cells survive to establish metastases elsewhere in the body. The bloodstream seems to be a particularly hostile environment for cancer cells. Even when particularly malignant cancer cells were injected into the blood of mice, only about 1 in 1000 were still alive 2 weeks later.[8] The immune system may destroy some of the wandering cancer cells, but clearly additional protective but unknown mechanisms are at work as well.

Metastases do not grow randomly throughout the body but

instead tend to occur in particular patterns.[9] Cancer of the breast most often metastasizes to the lungs, bones, liver, adrenal glands, and ovaries. Lung cancer often metastasizes to the brain. Cancers of the stomach metastasize to liver and lungs. Why cancer cells that originate in one tissue tend to metastasize only to certain other tissues is not known.

Cancers Kill in Many Ways

Cancers kill in ways that cannot always be precisely determined, and different cancers kill in different ways. In one study[10] done at a major cancer center, about 25 percent of all cancer deaths were the direct result of the growing mass of the cancer interfering with the function of an essential organ. Commonly, the immediate cause of death was impaired function of the lungs, liver, brain, or kidneys. Another 10 percent of cancer deaths resulted from severe emaciation (starvation). Some 7 percent resulted from hemorrhage, a frequent cause of death in leukemia; the disease impairs the blood's ability to form clots, and internal bleeding occurs readily and persists. By far the most common cause of death—accounting for about half of all cancer deaths in the study—is from bacterial infection. Bacteria that normally are killed by the immune system of a healthy individual can cause fatal infections in cancer victims. The lowered resistance to infecting bacteria partly results from the generally weak condition of a person with advanced cancer but is probably more the result of impaired immune defenses. For reasons that we do not understand, some cancers severely suppress the immune system (Chapter 10). Whatever the immediate cause of death, death by cancer is usually preceded by metastases and the establishment of secondary cancers.

Cancers Form Only
from Cells that Are Able to Divide

Cancers occur in different forms in different tissues and organs and often develop in different forms even in a single tissue. Cancers arise from almost any of the many kinds of cells in an organism and exhibit rates of development and degrees of malignancy that vary widely. In a very real sense, cancers may be thought of as a large family of related diseases with perhaps more than 100 varieties in all. Superficially various kinds of cancers do not seem to resemble one another: leukemia and lung cancer seem to have little in common, nor is there any obvious similarity between skin cancer and cancer of the pancreas. There are, nevertheless, underlying commonalities.

We have already discussed a few features common to all hundred or so kinds of cancers: features that relate to the failure of regulation of reproduction and differentiation at the cellular level. Another, related feature common to all cancers is their development in tissues that normally undergo at least some cell turnover or in tissues that retain the capacity to resume cell reproduction in the adult (e.g., skin, blood-forming tissues, major abdominal organs, and gonads). The common feature is the capacity to resume cell division, even if only rarely. Moreover, it appears that the transformation of a normal cell into a cancer cell is somehow associated with the process of cell division. Tissues that relinquish the capacity to resume cell division—nerve cells, cells of the voluntary muscles, and muscle cells of the heart—are virtually immune to cancer.[11]

Cancers apparently can result from exposure to a wide range of different agents, a topic that will be considered at length in later chapters. Cancers are known to be caused by a variety of chemicals (including inorganic compounds and simple and complex organic compounds), by ionizing radiations (such as X rays), by nonionizing radiations (such as ultraviolet rays in sunlight), by emissions from radioactive materials, and in animals generally and probably in humans, by viruses. A single form of cancer can be caused by several different agents, and a given agent may under some circumstances cause many different kinds of cancers. Yet, a common feature can be inferred here, too, namely, that most known cancer-causing agents are also known to cause mutations. Conversely, many agents that cause mutations are also capable of causing cancer. The inference is that most cancers arise through mutations or in the case of viruses, through changes in regulation of genes (see Chapter 9). Many lines of evidence support the inference that mutations are the basis of cancer. This evidence is presented in later chapters.

How might a mutation transform a normal cell into a malignant one? Although we have many clues, this difficult area of cancer research consists of more hypotheses than understanding. A variety of experiments that are described in detail in Chapter 3 suggest that normal cells stop dividing in response to regulatory signals, either internal or external. Experiments also suggest that this response requires the functions of at least a few genes, regulatory genes. It is not known how such regulatory genes might act to control cell reproduction, but if the function of one such regulatory gene were impaired by mutation, the cell might no longer respond appropriately to "stop" signals. Such a mutation would result in a line of cells that reproduce without limit—one of the characteristics of cancer cells.

Other characteristics of cancer cells suggest another feature of the possible genetic defect that underlies cancer. Cancer cells that produce rapidly and tend to metastasize readily (and thus are more malignant) also are generally poorly differentiated. In appearance and in behavior, such cells appear to be less mature, less developed than their normal counterparts. Conversely, cancer cells that reproduce less rapidly and metastasize more slowly (and are less malignant also are generally more highly differentiated. These observations along with others suggest that the reproduction and differentiation of each normal cell is controlled by regulatory genes, some of which act early in a genetically controlled pathway of differentiation and others later.

New cells in a tissue generally arise by division of so-called stem cells (Figure 5). STEM CELLS, themselves relatively undifferentiated, give rise to cells that ultimately differentiate into cells of the particular tissue the stem cells serve. When a stem cell divides, one daughter cell, on the average, remains a stem cell and the other begins to differentiate along a genetically programmed sequence of changes in structure and function. Differentiation is usually a gradual process involving many steps and occurs over several, or many, cell generations. The

STEM CELL

MUTATIONS

REPEATED CELL DIVISIONS

Poorly differentiated, malfunctional cells that grow rapidly and are immortal

HIGHLY MALIGNANT CANCER; RAPID METASTASES

MUTATIONS

REPEATED CELL DIVISIONS

Partly differentiated, poorly specialized cells with intermediate growth rates and long life spans (or immortal)

MODERATELY MALIGNANT CANCER; SLOW METASTASES

MUTATIONS

REPEATED CELL DIVISIONS

Well-differentiated cells with some specialized functions and nearly normal life spans and growth rates

WEAKLY MALIGNANT CANCER; VERY SLOW METASTASES

DIFFERENTIATION

Fully differentiated cells with specialized functions, fixed life spans, and slow (or no) growth

NORMAL TISSUE

◄ FIGURE 5   Differentiation of normal and abnormal progeny of a single stem cell. Branched lines represent successive cell divisions, with the normal pathway of differentiation represented from the top (original stem cell) to the bottom of the figure (normal differentiated tissue). Cancer-causing mutations (wavy arrows) disrupt the normal developmental sequence and lead to abnormal cell lines that differ in their degrees of specialization and growth rates (right side). In general, the more differentiated the cells in a cancer, the less malignant it will be.

process can be regarded as a developmental pathway of the kind illustrated in Figure 5. All along the pathway the differentiating cells continue to change gradually and to reproduce. These changes involve altered expression of the cells' genetic program but no change in the program itself. All of the progeny of each differentiating cell continue along the same pathway, following the same genetic program. The rate at which differentiating cells reproduce generally slows as successive generations proceed along the pathway. In this way, a single stem cell can give rise to many cells that all differentiate to replace cells lost from a particular tissue. When these cells reach the end of the differentiation pathway, they begin to perform normal functions of that tissue. They also stop dividing.

A mutation in a regulatory gene that acts early in the differentiation pathway may block the further differentiation of the cell that sustained the mutation.[12] The result is that the cell remains poorly differentiated throughout its life and continues to reproduce at the rate characteristic for a cell at that point in the pathway. All of its descendants will have these same properties. Thus, a mutation in a gene that acts early in the pathway may result in a line of poorly differentiated, rapidly growing, cells that form a highly malignant tumor (Figure 5). Similarly, mutations in late-acting regulatory genes might lead to slower-growing cancers made up of cells that had progressed further along their normal genetically controlled programs. These cancer cells would be more highly differentiated, more mature, and less malignant. This indeed is the pattern clinicians and researchers observe, supporting but not proving the ideas that controls over reproduction and over differentiation are somehow connected and that mutations may affect both processes in ways that result in the conversion of a normal cell into a cancer cell. The model also accounts for the fact that cancers arising in the same tissue may vary greatly in degree of differentiation and malignancy of their component cells.

It is thus a major task of cancer research to explain how and why normal controls over cell growth, reproduction, and differentiation sometimes become deranged. It is the contention of many, if not most, researchers that only on the basis of such knowledge will we understand the causes of cancer and how to prevent cancers or to develop more effective treatments. However, to understand the loss of controls in cancer requires first an understanding of virtually every aspect of the cell: there is simply no certain way to know in advance which feature(s) will turn out to be the critical one(s). In particular, it is necessary to understand the steps by which cells grow, reproduce, and differentiate. In addition, to understand how control over these processes may fail requires that we understand how the control systems normally operate. Basic research in the field of cell biology thus appears to be crucial for an adequate understanding of cancer. For this reason we consider next some fundamentals of cell biology.

3

The Reproduction
of Cells

ONE of the great generalizations of cell biology is the principle that the cells of higher organisms are all fundamentally similar, be they from plants or animals, normal or cancerous. There are, however, certain detailed differences that almost always enable us to identify cancer cells. Structural differences are particularly evident when cancer cells are compared microscopically with their normal counterparts from the tissue in which the cancer originated. Frequently, cancer cells occur as disorganized groups of cells, the disorganization being especially apparent against the background of the highly ordered and regular arrangement of normal cells in the same tissue (Figure 1). Pathologists search for such groups of abnormal cells as they examine potentially diseased tissues.

The really important differences between normal cells and cancer cells are functional and are reflected in the behavior of cancer cells, individually and as components of tissues and organs. As we have pointed out, cancer cells overproduce, do not differentiate or function normally, invade surrounding tissues, and crowd out normal cells. In Chapter 4 we will discuss the underlying bases of these characteristics that make cancer cells malignant. In this chapter, we describe the life histories of normal and cancerous cells, beginning with an overview of their structure and organization.[2]

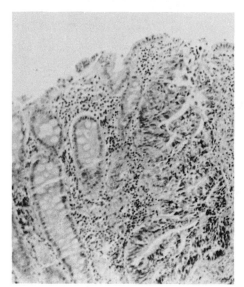

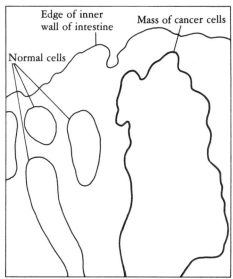

FIGURE 1   Light micrograph of a portion of a human large intestine showing normal and cancer cells. The intestine's hollow interior is at the top of the micrograph. Normal secretory cells (left) are elongated with many clear areas. Cells of an adenocarcinoma (right) form a poorly defined mass. The numerous dark spots outside the cells are the nuclei of lymphocytes.[1]

Normal and Cancerous Cells Are Structurally Similar

The cells of multicellular organisms are divided into two main compartments. The larger compartment, the CYTOPLASM, completely encloses the other main compartment, the NUCLEUS (Figures 2 and 3). Each of these main compartments contains a number of constituent parts or ORGANELLES that carry out different functions. The following is a brief account of the principal structures of a typical mammalian cell and their respective functions. Figures 2 and 4 illustrate many of the structures mentioned in the following paragraphs.

The cytoplasm is enclosed by an extremely thin PLASMA MEMBRANE, which separates the cell from its outside environment. The plasma membrane is too thin to be studied in detail with conventional microscopes, but the structure of plasma membranes can be observed by means of very great resolution provided by transmission electron miscroscopes (Figure 4). This thin membrane holds the cell together and prevents the *free* movement of molecules into and out of the cell. Molecules do constantly move across the plasma membrane but in a closely regulated way. Nutrients needed to support the life of a cell are moved from the surrounding medium into the cell's interior, and wastes are moved in the opposite direction—both

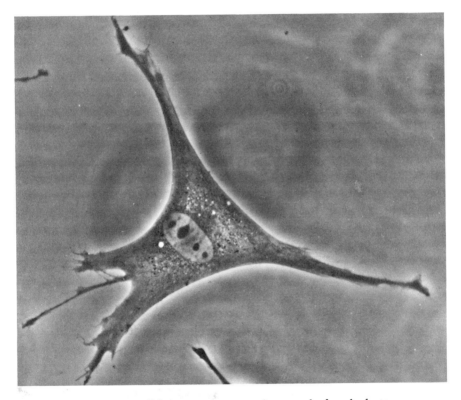

FIGURE 2   A living cell from a mouse, growing attached to the bottom of a culture dish containing a solution of nutrients. The relatively clear nuclear area is separated from the granular cytoplasm by a nuclear membrane that is not visible in this light micrograph. Within the nucleus are several dense nucleoli. The cell membrane, which encloses the cytoplasm and separates the cell from its surroundings, also cannot be seen in this micrograph.[3]

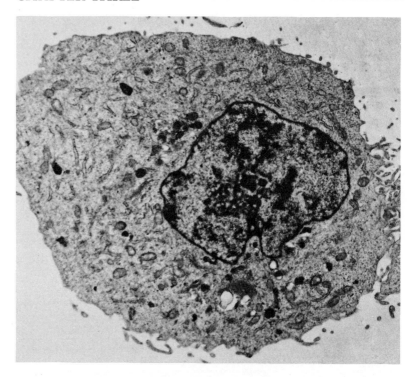

FIGURE 3 Electron micrograph of a section through a rat kidney cell grown in culture. The nucleus is outlined by a dark line, the nuclear membrane, and contains patches of dark material that are actually the fibrous chromosomes seen in section. The cytoplasm contains a variety of membranes and other cytoplasmic organelles.[4]

across the same membrane. A great deal of research has begun to reveal how the chemistry and organization of the plasma membrane regulate this traffic.

Details of the topography of cell surfaces, particularly of cells growing in cultures, can best be seen with scanning electron microscopes (Figure 5). The surfaces of cultured cells are covered with hundreds of minute projections. In addition, the cell's edges are ruffled at regions of active cell movement. Cells in culture, as well as many kinds of normal cells and most kinds of cancer cells in the body, use these ruffles as one way to move about.

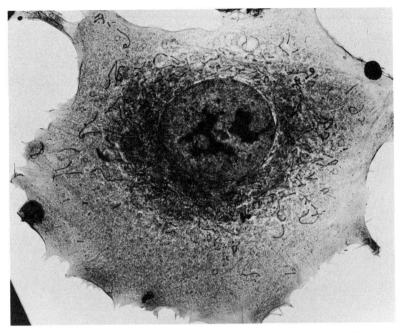

FIGURE 4   Electron micrograph of an entire rat kidney cell taken with the high voltage electron microscope at the University of Colorado at Boulder. In the center of the cell is the round nucleus. Surrounding the nucleus is the cell's cytoplasm, which contains a variety of structures, most apparent of which are the many thread-like mitochondria. Millions of ribosomes are partly responsible for the granular appearance of the cytoplasm. Enclosing the cytoplasm is the plasma membrane which, like the membrane enclosing the nucleus, is so thin as to be barely visible.[5]

Within the cytoplasmic compartment is an assortment of organelles, each of which performs a particular set of functions. MITOCHONDRIA (Figure 4) are small sacs in the cytoplasm that are often called the cell's "powerhouses." There may be up to a thousand or more in particularly active cells. Mitochondria contain enzymes that break down small molecules formed when carbohydrates and other energy-containing nutrients are digested in the cytoplasm. Other mitochondrial enzymes couple the breakdown of these small molecules to the formation of

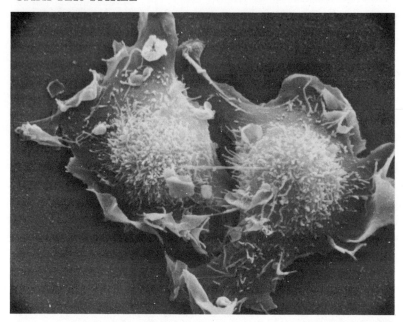

FIGURE 5 Scanning electron micrograph of two sarcoma cells from a rat. The surfaces of the cells are covered with numerous finger-like projections called microvilli. Their significance is not known. The ruffles around the edges of the cells are areas of active movement.[6]

new chemical bonds that trap energy in a form that can be stored and later used to drive energy-requiring activities in other parts of the cell. These energy-requiring activities include construction of large molecules from small ones, moving the cell and its contents, and exchanging nutrients and wastes across the plasma membrane.

The cytoplasm also contains an extensive array of membranes that form a network of interconnected channels collectively called the ENDOPLASMIC RETICULUM. These membranes, which can be resolved only with an electron microscope, perform a variety of functions including the channeling of newly synthesized proteins that are to be exported from the cell. The endoplasmic reticulum of some cells may also perform more specialized functions. In liver cells, for example, the endoplasmic reticulum contains enzymes that detoxify certain drugs and poisons, such as ethyl alcohol and barbiturates, that may be taken into the body.

Another specialized, smaller group of membranes and sacs, called the GOLGI APPARATUS, functions in the packaging of materials to be exported from the cell, for example, digestive enzymes produced by pancreas cells for export into the intestine.

Other cytoplasmic organelles called LYSOSOMES, smaller than mitochondria, are sacs of digestive enzymes enclosed in membranes formed by the Golgi body. These sacs fuse with other membrane-bound sacs that form when cells engulf bacteria and other kinds of particles; the enzymes of the lysosomes digest the engulfed particles. In healthy cells, the lysosomal membrane prevents the digestive enzymes stored in the lysosome from digesting the cell itself. However, when a cell dies, the lysosome's membrane breaks, and the released enzymes digest the components of the dead cell.

RIBOSOMES are extremely small particles within the cytoplasm and can be visualized only with the high resolution provided by electron microscopes. The ribosomes, of which there are many thousands in each cell, are the sites at which proteins are synthesized. Ribosomes may float free in the cytoplasm or they may be attached to the surfaces of endoplasmic reticulum.

All the organelles float in a complex water solution that contains many kinds of dissolved and suspended materials that carry out important cellular functions. In particular, many of the molecules in this solution act as messages and signals that coordinate and integrate the activities of the cell and its organelles.

These, then, are the main cellular components outside the nucleus of a typical mammalian cell: plasma membrane, mitochondria, endoplasmic reticulum, Golgi bodies, lysosomes, ribosomes, and the solution in which these float. Cells specialized for particular functions may contain other cytoplasmic structures: the cytoplasm of muscle cells is packed with contractile fibers; red blood cells contain large amounts of oxygen-carrying hemoglobin; plant cells have organelles known as chloroplasts, which carry out photosynthesis.

The other main compartment of a typical cell is the large

nucleus, which is separated from the cytoplasm by a NUCLEAR ENVELOPE (Figure 4). Also resolvable only with an electron microscope, the nuclear envelope is composed of *two* membranes flattened against one another. The nuclear envelope contains many pores that probably serve as routes for the movement of molecules between nucleus and cytoplasm.

A typical nucleus contains a well-defined organelle, the NUCLEOLUS (Figure 2); most nuclei contain two nucleoli, but there may be only one, or several. Large enough to be resolved with a conventional microscope, the nucleolus is the site in which ribosomes are constructed. From the nucleolus, ribosomes move through the nuclear envelope into the cytoplasm, where proteins are assembled on them.

Nuclei also contain CHROMOSOMES, which carry the cell's genetic program. Each chromosome is an enormously long but extremely thin molecule of DNA, which is the macromolecule that encodes genetic information (described in detail in Chapter 4). In a nondividing cell, these molecules twist and turn, snaking through the nucleus to form a complex meshwork of fibers (Figure 3). During cell division, the chromosomes coil up into shorter, well-defined bodies that can be resolved with conventional microscopes (Figure 6).

The number of chromosomes in the nuclei of body cells is a characteristic of each species. The *normal* chromosome number per cell is 26 in one species of frog; 44 in rabbits; 22 in the Chinese hamster; and 46 in humans (Figure 7A). The word "normal" is stressed because cancer cells usually contain extra chromosomes (Figure 7C).

The Life of a Cell
Can Be Described as a Cycle with Four Parts

When a cell divides, it forms two essentially identical daughter cells. The period between successive cell divisions is a convenient measure of a cellular generation, a cell's life span. Therefore, by definition, a cell's life span starts at the moment it separates from its sister cell at the instant cell division is completed and ends at the moment it divides to form two

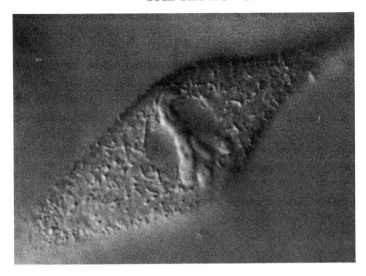

FIGURE 6   Photograph of a living cell taken from a rat kangaroo and grown in a culture vessel. In this cell, which is about to divide, the chromosomes have condensed into the large, rod-shaped structures in the cell's center. (Figure 11 shows the full course of events that chromosomes undergo during cell division.) The fine, threadlike objects in the cytoplasm are mitochondria.[7]

daughter cells (Figure 8). The end of life for one cell is thus the start of life for each of its two daughters. It is, however, more convenient here to represent a cell's life history as a cyclic process (rather than as the linear process presented in Figure 8), which begins and ends with newly formed cells (Figure 9). Although the cell that begins the cycle doesn't, strictly speaking, exist at the end of the cycle, its identical daughters do, and it is customary to speak of a CELL CYCLE.

In order for a newly formed cell to complete a cell cycle and reach the point of being ready to divide, it must complete a number of preparations. Some of these preparations occur in the cytoplasm, others are centered in the nucleus. Most of the cytoplasmic preparations result in the enlargement, the growth, of the cell. These include increases in the numbers and amounts of all cytoplasmic components (including endoplasmic reticu-

(A)

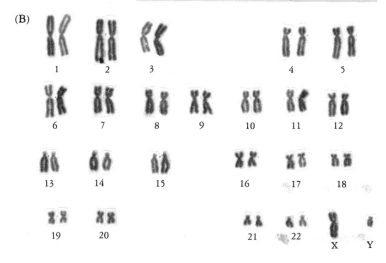

(B)

lum, mitochondria, ribosomes), as well as materials in the solution in which all of the components are suspended. Preparations that result in growth start at the beginning of the cell cycle (the bars in Figure 8) with the cell taking in raw materials from its surroundings. As time passes, these raw materials are converted into new cellular materials, and the cell grows and becomes larger. From the standpoint of growth, there is nothing to distinguish one part of the interval between divisions from another; growth progresses smoothly from division to division.

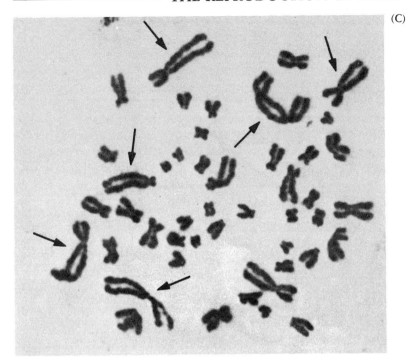

(C)

FIGURE 7   Chromosome complements from normal and cancerous human cells. (A) Light micrograph of the 46 fully condensed chromosomes from a normal cell. (B) These normal chromosomes arranged into 22 pairs plus an X and Y, signifying a male; cells from normal human females contain the corresponding 22 pairs plus two X chromosomes. (C) Light micrograph of condensed chromosomes from a human breast cancer cell. Arrows point to abnormal chromosomes.[8]

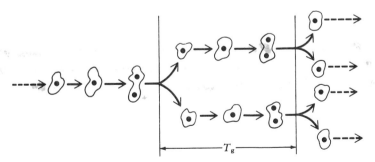

FIGURE 8 T_g, the generation time, defines the life span of a cell as the time between successive cell divisions.

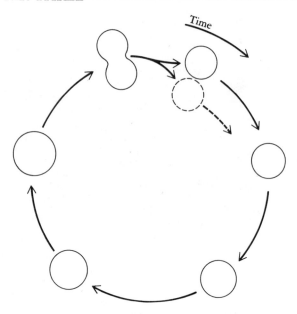

FIGURE 9   A cell's life history can be represented as a cycle.

Nuclear preparations for division consist mainly of the cell duplicating its chromosomes. When both sets of preparations are complete (that is, when the cell has doubled all of its parts, including its chromosomes), the actual division of the fully grown cell into two daughter cells begins.

One of the major tasks of cell biology, one that is especially relevant to the understanding of cancer, is to determine how cells accomplish these preparations for cell division and how cell division is started. Early studies resolved the cell cycle into a DIVISION PHASE during which the movements of chromosomes and the separation of daughter cells were readily observed and an INTERPHASE (a phase between divisions) during which only the gradual enlargement of the cell was obvious (Figure 9). More recent studies resolved both phases into sequences of coordinated processes, which then became the subjects of more detailed analyses.

Contemporary studies of the cell cycle center on efforts to

develop answers to a set of questions about cellular growth: What are the steps that result in the growth of a cell? How is each step accomplished? How are the various steps controlled and coordinated with one another? A similar set of questions centers on the process by which chromosomes duplicate: How are the cytoplasmic preparations coordinated with those in the nucleus? When all of the preparations for division are completed, what triggers the cell to divide into two cells? Continuing research is developing answers to these and other questions about the cell cycle that bear on the nature of cancer. It must, however, be admitted that neither the cell cycle nor cancer is yet well understood. The balance of this chapter and much of the next summarize contemporary understanding.

An important result of efforts to answer such questions is the resolution of the cycle into four periods that are defined by the key processes occurring in each (Figure 10). These periods occur in the cycles of all cells of higher organisms, including cancerous cells. Three of these periods are subdivisions of what was earlier known as the interphase: G1, S, and G2. The S refers to the period of DNA synthesis, which is the essential event of chromosome duplication. G1 and G2 are growth periods preceding and following the synthesis of DNA. D, the fourth period of the cell cycle, is, of course, the division phase itself.

For very rapidly reproducing human cells, the entire cycle occupies about 16 hours. Most cell types, including most cancer cells, have much longer generation times. In the case of a normal cell with a generation time of 16 hours, the G1 period occupies about 5 hours, the S period about 8 hours, G2 about 2 hours, and D about 1 hour. In a cancer cell with a generation time of about 16 hours, the durations of the four periods would be essentially identical; cancer cells rarely ever reproduce so rapidly in the body, although they may do so in a culture vessel. Coordination of the events in the four periods results in the distribution to each daughter cell of a full set of parental chromosomes and about half the parental cytoplasm and organelles. D, the period of cell division, is a convenient point for beginning a discussion of the details of the cell cycle.

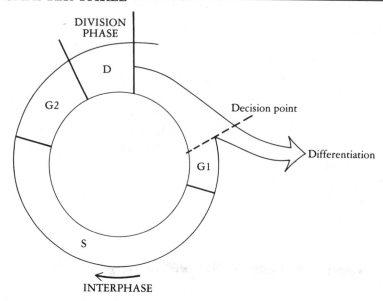

FIGURE 10   Outline of the cell cycle for a typical mammalian cell. A newly formed cell grows steadily until it divides, but it synthesizes DNA only during a period called the S phase. The entire cycle occupies at least 8 hours and typically lasts about 24 hours in adult tissues. G1 is the most variable phase, ranging up to hours or even days. Cells that no longer divide are permanently arrested in G1. Cells usually differentiate after becoming arrested in G1.

Cell Division Produces Genetically Identical Cells

Cell division actually consists of two processes: the division of the nucleus, called MITOSIS, and the division of the cytoplasm, called CYTOKINESIS. The first indication that a cell has entered the D period is detected in the nucleus. All during interphase (Figure 10; G1, S, and G2 combined), the chromosomes are so stretched out that they cannot be resolved by light microscopy. These threadlike chromosomes twist and bend as they course through the nucleus, creating a tangled, fibrous meshwork (Figure 11A). As division begins, each chromosome begins to coil up, much as a long piece of rope might be coiled into the shape of a long, thin spring (Figure 12). This coiling shortens the chromosome and makes it thicker. The coil itself then coils, condensing the chromosome still further.

Coiling continues until each chromosome is many times shorter and many times thicker than its interphase form. At the end of the condensation phase, each chromosome is a tightly packaged, rod-shaped structure that is clearly visible in the light microscope. In the fully condensed state, each chromosome has a characteristic size and shape that usually makes it distinguishable from the others. The 46 chromosomes of a normal human cell are shown in the fully condensed state in Figure 7; 20–25 minutes are required for human chromosomes to reach the state shown in this figure.

As the chromosomes approach the fully condensed state, the nuclear envelope disintegrates and the dividing cell comes to consist of a single large compartment containing all the cell's contents, including, of course, the condensed chromosomes. At about this time it becomes evident that each chromosome is, in fact, double [that is, each chromosome is composed of *two* condensed threads (Figure 11B)]. The doubleness of each predivision chromosome stems from the duplication of the chromosomes that occurred during the *prior* S period (Figure 10). Before the S period, a chromosome consists of a single thread; during the S period, each chromosome is duplicated, yielding a double thread. This duplication involves the formation of two DNA molecules from one, a process that will be described in Chapter 4. In any case, the two parts of each duplicated chromosome are initially attached to one another. Some minutes after the chromosomes reach the fully condensed state, all of the condensed chromosomes, each with the two daughter parts still attached to one another, quickly become arranged at the equator of the cell (Figure 11C). The chromosomes are positioned so that one half of each doubled chromosome faces one side of the parental cell and the other half faces the opposite side. Next the doubled chromosomes split into halves nearly simultaneously, producing paired daughter chromosomes (Figure 11D). All of the daughter chromosomes facing one direction form a group that moves away from its sister group. This movement of the two groups of daughter chromosomes continues for a few minutes until the two groups reach opposite sides of the dividing cell (Figure 11E).

As the daughter chromosomes are moving apart, a furrow

(A)

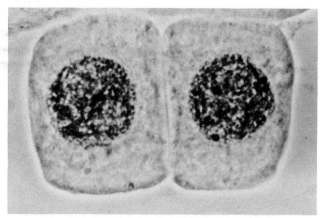

(B)

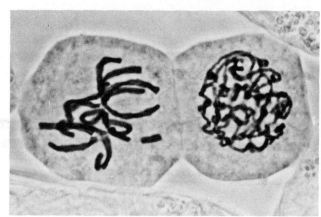

(C)

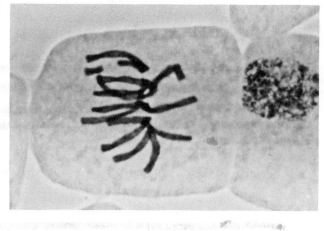

(D)

(E)

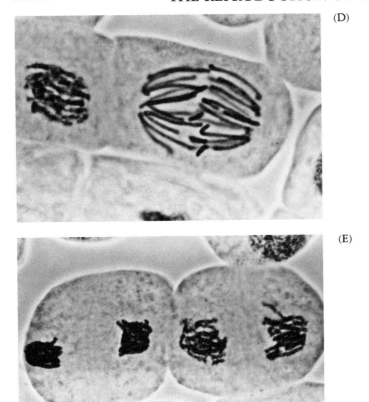

FIGURE 11   Mitosis in cells from the tips of bean root, particularly favorable material for observing details of this process. (A) Two cells during interphase with threadlike chromosomes tangled together. In the stage shown here (G2), the chromosomes have already replicated. The nuclear membranes, not visible in this image, are still intact. (B) Two cells early in mitosis. In both, the chromosomes are condensing and untangling, processes that have progressed further in the cell to the left. (C) Fully condensed chromosomes line up across the cell's equator (oriented vertically here), then (D) separate so that one full set of chromosomes passes to each pole of the cell. (E) Two cells late in mitosis. In each, cell walls are starting to form across the equator (vertical here). Nuclear membranes will also form around the decondensing chromosomes, resulting in two daughter cells from each original. This final stage is somewhat different in animal cells, as described in the text.[9]

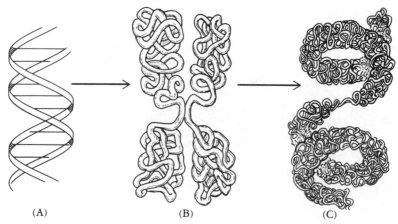

(A)   (B)   (C)

FIGURE 12   A model that accounts for many features of the ways DNA folds and coils in the chromosomes of higher organisms. (A) A portion of a DNA helix. (B) Coiling of the kind that occurs in chromosomes during metaphase of mitosis. The fibers are coiled-up helices. (C) In some species, metaphase chromosomes of the kind shown in B coil still another time.

forms at the equator of the cell's surface. This cleavage furrow rapidly deepens, so that in a few minutes the cell has been split into two parts, each of which contains a full set of daughter chromosomes. During this time the daughter chromosomes in each new cell start to decondense—a reversal of the condensation that took place as the parental cell entered the D period. Decondensation is completed within a few minutes after the daughter cells separate, returning the chromosomes to the interphase form of finely dispersed threads (Figure 11A). A nuclear envelope is quickly formed around the set of decondensing chromosomes in each daughter cell, completing the formation of new daughter nuclei. The D period ends a few minutes later when the daughter chromosomes are fully decondensed. Each daughter cell is then ready to enter a new cell cycle at G1, and they begin to grow in preparation for the next duplication of chromosomes and the subsequent division.

To recapitulate, then, the D period begins when the parental chromosomes, which had been duplicated in the previous S period (Figure 10), condense into tight packages. Each of the condensed, doubled chromosomes splits in two to form identical daughter chromosomes, which become aligned across the cell's equator. Sets of daughter chromosomes then move as two groups to opposite poles, and the parental cell splits into two daughter cells. In each daughter cell, the chromosomes decondense and are enclosed in a nuclear envelope. Each of the two resulting daughter cells is then ready to enter a new cell cycle. Thus, by a smooth progression of events, a cell divides into two identical cells each of which receives about half of the cytoplasm and organelles of the parental cell and exactly one full set of chromosomes that are identical to those of the parental cell. Identical sets of chromosomes do, of course, carry identical genetic programs. That is the essence of the cell cycle: to maintain genetic continuity across time (see Chapter 4 for details). Explaining these events in molecular terms is a formidable task, but recent progress toward this important objective has been substantial.

The condensation–decondensation of chromosomes during cell division is an efficient way to accomplish the orderly distribution of chromosomes to daughter cells. As we will suggest in Chapter 4, the functions of the chromosomes during G1 and G2 and their duplication during S probably require that the chromosomes be in the highly extended interphase state (Figure 11A). During the G1 period, the DNA molecule in an average human chromosome is about 1.25 inches (3 cm) long. Forty-six such chromosomes are contained in a roughly spherical nucleus with a maximum diameter of about 1/5000 of an inch (5 μm). Thus, the DNA molecule in an average chromosome is about 5000 times longer than the maximum dimension of the space in which it is contained. We can put the matter into more familiar dimensions by enlarging each component by 100,000 times. On such a scale, a DNA molecule would be as thick as fine sewing thread (about 1/100 of an inch or 0.25 mm thick) and almost 2 miles (3.2 km) long. A cell's nucleus increased in the same proportion would have a diameter of 2.5 feet (75 cm). The sorting out of 46 fine threads, each 2 miles long, all inside an envelope 2.5 feet in diameter, would seem an insurmountable task.

Obviously, the separation and movement of the chromosomes will be far less complicated if they are tightly packaged than if they remain extended. The coiling of the chromosomes into tight packages may also serve to disentangle the two duplicated halves of a chromosome from each other and from other chromosomes so that they can separate and move to the daughter cells efficiently. Uncoiling near the end of the D period restores the daughter chromosomes to the functional interphase state.

Although the means by which a cell divides itself into two daughter cells also may seem complex at first, it is difficult to imagine a simpler scheme for achieving the same ends. The processes of the D period not only work, but they work rapidly and extremely efficiently. In the adult human about 10 million cells divide every second, and mistakes or misfunctions are extremely rare. Errors consist mostly in the failure of chromosomes to split into daughter chromosomes, failure of daughter chromosomes to move apart correctly, or failure of the cell to divide itself into equal halves. No accurate measure of the frequency of such mistakes in living human tissue is available; however, judging from the number of errors detected in normal human cells growing and dividing in culture, the frequency of abnormal cell divisions is extremely small.[10]

The division period (D) ends when two genetically identical daughter cells are created. These begin to traverse the interphase of the next cell cycle, entering the G1 period (Figure 10). The activities accomplished during G1 vary for different kinds of cells. Cells programmed to differentiate to specialized functions do so during the G1 period and may remain arrested in this part of the cycle as long as they live. Cells whose fate it is to reproduce will grow during G1 as they also prepare for and progress toward the next S period. The duration of these activities varies for cells of different tissues, as you will see in the next section. G1 ends and the S period begins when the cell begins to duplicate its DNA chromosomes. Growth continues throughout the S period into the G2 period. During the G2 period, which separates the end of DNA duplication from the beginning of cell division, the cell continues to grow as it prepares for division. As described earlier, cell division begins with division of the nucleus and ends with the division of the cytoplasm.

This separation of the cell cycle into periods labeled G1, S, G2, and D is a convenience employed by biologists to facilitate their descriptions and analyses of the growth events and reproduction of a typical cell. Each period, however, includes a multitude of events and processes, few of which are fully understood. These are exquisitely coordinated, with the completion of one step tied to and integrated with subsequent steps. The study of this progression of the cell cycle is widely thought to be the key to understanding how both normal and cancer cells reproduce and also to be the key to determining how and why the reproduction and differentiation of cancer cells are out of control.

Cell Reproduction Is Regulated by Delaying or Stopping Cells in G1

As mentioned in Chapter 2, very few types of cells reproduce at the maximum possible rate within the body. Rather, in tissues that turn over, a close balance is maintained between the rate at which normal cells differentiate and die and the rate at which they are replaced through cell division. The rate at which a cell does reproduce is regulated by interrupting or stopping its progress through the cell cycle. This interruption is accomplished in a rather specific way as suggested by Table 1. For most kinds of cells, the durations of S, G2, and D periods tend to be fairly constant no matter how long the cell cycle. The length of the cell cycle seems to be controlled mostly by regulating the duration of the G1 period. In cells that reproduce very rapidly (e.g., the blood-producing cells of the bone marrow), the G1 period is on the order of a few hours. In slowly reproducing liver cells, by contrast, the G1 period is more than 400 *days* long. In the extreme situation of cells reproducing at the maximum possible rate, the duration of the G1 period may be virtually zero. The only way in which progress through the cell cycle could be further accelerated would be to shorten one or more of the other three periods of the

TABLE 1. Approximate durations of periods of the cell cycle for some representative cell types.[10]

Cell Type	Duration of Period (Hours)				
	Entire Cycle	G1	S	G2	D
Blood-forming marrow	$\cong 13$	2	8	2	0.7
Ileum	$\cong 17$	6	8	2	0.7
Duodenum	$\cong 18$	7	8	2	0.7
Colon	$\cong 33$	22	8	2	0.7
Tongue	$\cong 40$	28	8	3	0.7
Esophagus	$\cong 181$	170	8	2	0.7
Skin	$\cong 1,000$	989	8	2	0.7
Liver	$> 10,000$	$>9,989$	8	2	0.7
Mature nerve, muscle	(Do not divide beyond infancy)				

cycle. This ordinarily does not happen. The S, G2, and D periods are about the same whether a cell is reproducing rapidly or slowly, suggesting that processes accomplished in each of these periods cannot be accelerated—at least not as a means to shorten the cell cycle.

The idea that the duration of G1 determines the duration of the cell cycle comes from several different observations. One is that cells that normally do not divide contain the same amount of DNA as newly formed cells. So do cells that are capable of reproducing but happen not to be so engaged. Given that the amount of DNA per cell begins to increase at the start of S, doubles by the end of S, and remains at that level until the end of division, it is clear that cells pause only during G1. Another relevant observation comes from experiments in which cultured cells that have been dividing are deprived of an essential nutrient, say an amino acid. Some cells may continue to grow for a time, but all cells soon stop dividing. They do not resume dividing until the missing nutrient is resupplied. If the nutrient is withheld for the equivalent of a cell generation and then resupplied, all cells soon begin to synthesize DNA, that is, they resume the cell cycle at or near the transition from G1 to S.[10]

The essential point is that the rate of reproduction of each cell type is regulated by controlling the duration of the G1 period. Cells that reproduce very slowly have very long G1 periods; cells that reproduce at or near the maximum possible rate have very short G1 periods.

A clear example of cells dividing so rapidly that their cycles include virtually no G1 period comes from the earliest stages of embryological development. The cycles by which a fertilized egg and its immediate daughter cells divide have no G1 sections. This continues to be the case until eight or nine rounds of cell division produce a mass of several hundred cells. As development proceeds beyond this stage, the cell mass begins to resemble an embryo, with traces of an embryonic brain, spinal cord, heart, and muscles. At about that stage, the rate of cell reproduction of certain cell types begins to slow down, that is, to be regulated by the prolongation of the G1 periods. This programmed regulation of the G1 period, and thus of cell reproduction, ultimately results in cell cycles of characteristic lengths for each of the many embryonic cell types. Such regulation of cell reproduction is essential not only for normal embryonic development but for normal postnatal growth and development as well.[10]

In Chapter 2 we spoke of tissues that turn over and those that do not and noted that cancers arise only in tissues that do. We can now enlarge on that view by incorporating the variability of the G1 period. The rates of cell reproduction found in the different tissues cover a broad spectrum from the extremely high rate of bone marrow cells to the extremely low rates in liver, pancreas, and some other tissues. Under certain conditions the rates of reproduction can be drastically altered. For example, if a large part of the liver is removed, the reproduction of the remaining liver cells is enormously accelerated: the G1 period shortens from thousands of hours to only a few hours. That rate of cell reproduction replaces the missing liver tissue in a few days. At that time, the G1 period returns to the normal duration of 400 or so days so that the rate of reproduction falls to the normal low rate that matches the rate at which liver cells die.[10]

Thus, the duration of G1 is under flexible control: when

only a low rate of cell reproduction is required to maintain the health of a tissue, the cells remain arrested in G1 for a correspondingly long time; when rapid cell reproduction is needed, the G1 arrest is correspondingly shorter.

Normally, the cell cycle is interrupted *only* in the G1 period. Stopping a cell during the S period of its cycle, for example, by depriving it of an essential precursor of DNA, is usually lethal. This fact is the basis for an important approach to cancer chemotherapy, as you will see in Chapter 10. Occasionally, cells do stop in the G2 period, which suggests that a natural stopping point exists in G2, but this stopping point is infrequently used. Cell division can be interrupted with certain chemicals and in other ways, but normally division is not interrupted once it has started.

We can summarize all of the foregoing quite simply. The rate of cell reproduction is regulated by stopping a cell in the G1 period and holding it there for the appropriate period of time (Figure 13). Whatever the molecular mechanism by which regulation occurs, it operates by affecting some activity in the G1 period. This conclusion may seem vague, but it is nevertheless an important clue. It means that the key to understanding how cell division is controlled is to be sought among the particular events or activities that occur during the G1 period, that is, *prior* to the period of DNA duplication. *This also means that in whatever way a normal cell is converted to a cancer cell, the conversion must specifically disrupt the normal G1 arrest.*

Neither the key event that leads to G1 arrest nor the molecular basis for this phenomenon has yet been identified. However, there are good reasons to think that the key event on which matters hinge is related to the beginning of DNA duplication, that is, to the *transition from G1 to S*. The reasoning is as follows. At some (as yet unidentified) point in the G1 period, some (as yet unknown) events are set in motion that ultimately initiate the duplication of DNA. In other words, at some point during the G1 period a decision is made to proceed to the next round of DNA duplication, that is, to the next S period.

This decision to enter the S period without further pause is crucial because once the cell enters into preparations to

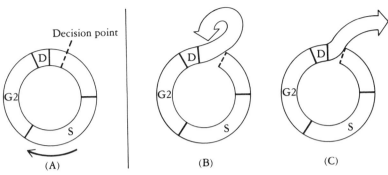

FIGURE 13   Variations on the basic cell cycle. (A) Cells that pass the decision point proceed to S, complete the cell cycle, and divide. (B) Cells that become arrested and (C) cells that begin to differentiate somehow avoid the G1 decision point, either temporarily (B) or permanently (C).

duplicate its DNA, it normally proceeds through the rest of the cell cycle, including cell division. Only by delaying the start of S can the G1 period be extended and the cell cycle regulated.

Each time a cell cycles through G1, the point of decision must be passed. By means that are unfortunately not known, normal cells are able to make correct decisions; they remain arrested at the decision point for precisely the appropriate time and thereby divide neither too infrequently nor too often. This capacity is as much a part of the normal program of differentiation as is the programmed death of normal cells. Cells programmed to turn over at characteristic rates seem to have characteristic periods of G1 arrest built into their programs. Cells that adjust their rates of division in response to external stimuli seem able to modify the G1 arrest program, making decisions about the transition from G1 to S responsively and flexibly. Such flexible responses are essential, for example, to accelerate cell reproduction in damaged tissues.

G1 Arrest Is Defective in Cancer Cells

At the end of cell division, each daughter cell enters the G1 period of the next cell cycle. Normal daughter cells then begin to synthesize new proteins and other materials and thus to grow larger. After some required amount of growth has occurred, a cell in a tissue that is turning over or repairing itself enters the S period by beginning to synthesize DNA. When the chromosomes are duplicated, the cell finishes its major preparations for division. Activities during the ensuing G2 period are only poorly documented, but in general the G2 period may be looked upon as the time required by the cell to arrange itself to divide during the subsequent D period of the cycle.

The cell cycles of cancer cells consist of G1, S, G2, and D periods that are directly comparable to the corresponding periods in normal cells. Moreover, in a cancer cell with a generation time of 16 hours, the duration of each period of the cycle will be about the same as in a normal cell with a generation time of 16 hours (for example, an intestinal cell). There is nothing about the sequence or timing of its cell cycle that distinguishes a cancer cell from a normal cell.[10]

A characteristic that does distinguish a cancer cell from its normal counterpart is the failure of a cancer cell to make appropriate decisions about the transition from G1 to S. More specifically, the capacity of a cancer cell to remain arrested in G1 is defective. Each kind of cancer cell grows at a characteristic rate that reflects the time spent in G1. For example, in certain kinds of leukemia, cancerous white blood cells may divide once every few days—much more often than their mature normal counterparts. In some cancers of the liver (hepatomas), on the other hand, cells may reproduce very slowly; indeed, the average cancer cell divides into two only once in many days but still far more rapidly than the mature normal counterpart. It is a perplexing attribute of cancer cells, however, that the defect in G1 arrest is rarely complete. Very few kinds of cancer cells reproduce at rates that would indicate that G1 arrest was completely eliminated. In the majority of cancers, cells continue to be retained in the G1 period; however, they do not progress to the fully differentiated form with its corresponding sharply reduced reproduction rate.

Another important point to remember from Chapter 2 is that cancer cells fail to differentiate normally. Differentiation

TABLE 2. A comparison of some important features of the cell cycles of normal and cancer cells.

Feature	Normal Cells	Cancer Cells
Regulation of reproduction	Controlled	Defective
Transition from G1 to S	Regulated	Poorly or not regulated
Differentiation	Normal	Abnormal
Life span	Die on schedule	Do not die on schedule; may be immortal

almost always includes a reduced rate of reproduction, the acquisition of specialized functions, and programmed death. Cancer cells, unable to regulate G1 arrest normally, continue to reproduce when their normal counterparts have differentiated and slowed down or stopped reproduction. A defect that leads to cancer usually results in the incessant and relentless reproduction of incompletely differentiated, malfunctioning cells that are often immortal (Table 2 and Figure 5 in Chapter 2).

Much current basic research in cell biology seeks to understand the means by which the reproduction and differentiation of normal cells are so precisely regulated. Much current research on cancer seeks to understand how and why the reproduction and differentiation of cancer cells are defective. Accordingly, it is of utmost importance to bring to light the molecular nature of the events that control the transition from G1 to S, that is, the initiation of DNA duplication. An understanding of this crucial step will probably provide new insights into the normal mechanism for controlling cell reproduction. Insight into the control mechanism is, in turn, likely to yield insights into the central molecular defect(s) in cancer cells. Identifying the defect is considered by many researchers as the only means by which to develop new, more highly effective anticancer tools. Because of the central position of DNA in this analysis of the cancer problem, we devote the next chapter to an explanation of the replication of this essential molecule.

4

The Genetic Basis
of Cancer

ARLIER chapters have established that cancer is transmitted from cell to cell through cell division. In particular, the conversion of a normal cell to the cancerous state consists of a heritable defect in the normal controls over a cell's reproduction and differentiation. This chapter explores further the nature of this defect and the connections between genetics and cancer.

Perhaps the most obvious clue to the genetic basis of cancer is the observation that every descendant of a cancer cell is itself a cancer cell. Another important fact established beyond question is that cancer can be caused by various kinds of radiation and by certain chemicals. The kinds of radiation that cause cancer and many of the chemicals that cause cancer are also efficient inducers of permanent genetic changes; that is, they cause mutations (Chapters 7 and 8). It is also likely that viruses cause some human cancers, also by altering a cell's genetic makeup (Chapter 9). Finally, susceptibility to certain kinds of cancer runs in families, both in humans and in laboratory animals (Chapter 5), demonstrating hereditary factors in the susceptibility to cancer.

These and other observations about cancer and its causes lead to a fundamentally important generalization: the conversion of a normal cell to a cancer cell is the result of a MUTATION, a permanent genetic change in that cell. This concept of the mutational basis of cancer underlies much of the modern study of cancer and is a central theme of this book. Experiments and experiences that support this view are presented in subsequent chapters. The basics of molecular genetics are outlined in this chapter, providing an important background for later chapters.[1]

Each Gene Directs the Formation of a Unique Protein

Every cell contains hundreds of thousands of protein molecules. All of the structures in a cell, such as ribosomes, fibers, and the many membranes that delimit the nucleus, mitochondria, endoplasmic reticulum, and other cellular compartments, are composed at least in part of proteins.

Many other proteins are enzymes, which guide and control the chemical changes that go on within the cell. Enzymes act by speeding up the many chemical reactions that cells perform, reactions that would otherwise happen too slowly to sustain life. The sum of all the chemical changes that occur in a cell produces the particular behaviors observed for that cell. The conduction of nerve impulses, the contraction of muscle cells, the ameboid movement of white blood cells, and the absorption of nutrients by intestinal cells are all the results of enzymatic activities of various proteins.

Some cells make proteins that they then export. One of the functions of liver cells is to produce certain proteins that make up part of the serum of blood. Most of the cells of the pancreas produce proteins that are released into a duct that carries them to the small intestine where the proteins act as digestive enzymes. Other cells of the pancreas produce the protein hormone, insulin.

All cells constantly make new protein molecules to replace protein molecules that wear out or are otherwise lost. Some protein molecules have life spans of only a few hours, most last at least a few days, and others may last for months. In any event, every cell must produce thousands of proteins every minute to maintain its functional integrity. Finally, to grow and reproduce, a cell must double its content of proteins as it proceeds through the cell cycle from one division to the next.

One of this century's major milestones in biology was the recognition that the information needed to produce individual proteins is carried in the cell's chromosomes. We now know that each chromosome consists of a series of genes arranged in a linear order and that each gene directs the formation of a particular protein. Considered together, a cell's complement of genes is like a set of blueprints that contains all the information and instructions needed for the cell to grow, reproduce, and differentiate. Every normal cell of a person's body contains a full set of chromosomes within which are distributed a full set of genes. In a given cell, however, only a fraction of the complement of genes is likely to be in use at a given moment. The fraction of the genes being used determines the behavior and features of that cell, just as using a portion of a set of blueprints leads to the construction of a particular part of a building.

Some genes are "read," or expressed, most of the time in most cells, for example, genes concerned with the normal repair and maintenance of a cell's membrane. Other genes are active only under special circumstances or in response to specific signals. For example, cells of the mammary gland respond to the hormone prolactin by activating genes concerned with synthesis of the proteins of milk. Finally, some genes may never be expressed in a given type of cell. The development of a fertilized egg into a multicellular organism involves the specialization of genetically identical cells. This specialization, or differentiation, comes about as different parts of the gene complement are selectively activated or silenced in different cells. Cells that differentiate into liver cells do so by activating a number of genes that are silenced in cells that differentiate into skin or into blood-forming tissues. Similarly, in a differentiating skin cell, genes that would be active in liver or blood cells are silenced. Therefore, although each cell contains a copy of every gene, some genes are selectively activated and others are selectively inactivated as each cell type differentiates. That is the essence of differentiation.

This selective activation of a cell's genes determines many features of the structure and behavior of a cell by determining which of the many proteins the cell is able to make are actually made, when they are made, and in what amounts. The gene complement of a normal human cell, for example, can specify the formation of thousands of different proteins. Some of these are proteins that form part of the substance of the cellular and nuclear membranes and of the membranes that define organelles such as mitochondria and the endoplasmic reticulum. Other proteins form fibers such as the contractile fibers of muscle.

The means by which genes are inactivated and either kept that way or reactivated is not understood, although important clues come from studies with bacteria and viruses. An understanding of these processes is important both in its own right and as a clue to the genetic basis of cancer, because among the genes that may be activated or inactivated in a particular cell are those that normally control the duplication of the genes themselves. In normal cells, control of cell division is achieved by preventing the duplication of the chromosomes. In cancer cells, the duplication proceeds, inadequately controlled, apparently because genes that should be silenced are not.

Proteins are large polymers (macromolecules), each made up of from 100 to 500 building blocks (subunits), depending on the particular protein. There are 20 different kinds of subunits, collectively called the AMINO ACIDS (Figure 1). Each kind of protein macromolecule consists of a chain of amino acid subunits linked together in a specific sequence (Figure 2). Each amino acid has characteristic physical and chemical properties; some are larger than others, or more soluble in water, or carry positive or negative electrical charges. It is the side groups of the amino acids (Figure 1) that determine these characteristics, and these side groups can interact with one another in various ways. Such interactions follow the laws of chemistry and make possible the variety and specificity of proteins. These interactions cause the linear chain of amino acids to fold up into a three-dimensional shape that is characteristic for each sequence of amino acids, each kind of protein. Whatever the pattern of folding, it is precisely determined by the interactions among the side groups of the particular sequence of amino acids in that protein. The three-dimensional geometry, in turn, gives the protein its particular functional ability.

The number of theoretically possible sequences of amino acids and therefore the number of theoretically possible proteins is immense. However, a cell can produce a given protein only if it contains a gene that specifies the appropriate sequence of amino acids, and then only if that gene is active. Thus, the link between a cell's genes and its properties and behavior is through the proteins it makes. The link is indirect and a little complicated, involving other kinds of macromolecules. First, however, it will be helpful to examine the chemical nature of genes and the chemistry of how genes duplicate themselves.

A Gene Is a Segment of a DNA Macromolecule

Research during the 1940s and 1950s demonstrated that genetic information for assembling proteins is carried in enormously long macromolecules called DEOXYRIBONUCLEIC ACIDS or DNAs. This recognition was one of the great intellectual achievements of the twentieth century; it reshaped thinking about biology in general and about the biology of cells in particular.[2]

Like proteins, DNAs are polymers composed of subunits connected in a linear sequence—a property of considerable significance, as becomes clear later in this chapter. Individual nucleic acids are called POLYNUCLEOTIDES because they consist of many NUCLEOTIDE subunits. The nucleotides are, in turn, assembled from three smaller building blocks: a phosphate, a sugar, and an organic base (Figure 3). The phosphate building block is the same in all nucleic acids, but the sugar and organic base portions differ among the kinds of nucleic acids. DNAs contain the sugar deoxyribose and the organic bases abbreviated as T, A, G, and C below and in Figure 4. The other class of nucleic acids, the RIBONUCLEIC ACIDS or RNAs, whose function is explained later, contains the sugar ribose and the bases U, A, G, and C. Nucleic acids of both classes contain the same kind of phosphate group. Together the sugar–phosphate groups form the backbone of a polynu-

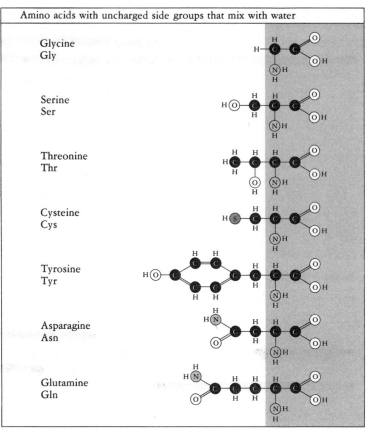

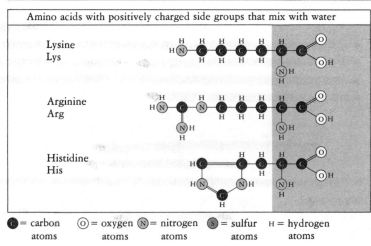

= carbon atoms = oxygen atoms = nitrogen atoms = sulfur atoms H = hydrogen atoms

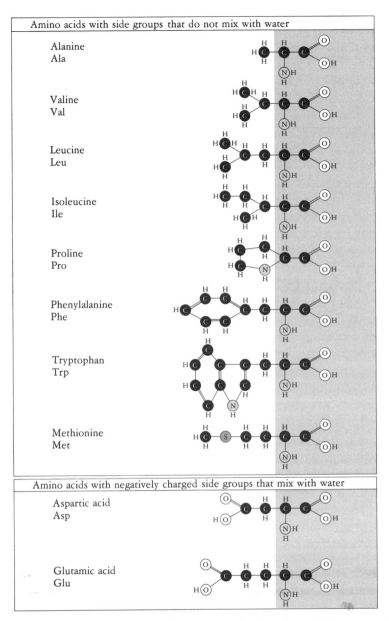

Amino acids with side groups that do not mix with water

Alanine
Ala

Valine
Val

Leucine
Leu

Isoleucine
Ile

Proline
Pro

Phenylalanine
Phe

Tryptophan
Trp

Methionine
Met

Amino acids with negatively charged side groups that mix with water

Aspartic acid
Asp

Glutamic acid
Glu

FIGURE 1 The 20 amino acids from which polypeptides are assembled. Each amino acid has a unique cluster of atoms that accounts for its particular properties. These SIDE GROUPS may or may not mix with water; if they mix, they may be positively or negatively charged, or neutral. Nineteen of the 20 amino acids share a common cluster of atoms that account for the common properties of amino acids as a group (the exception is proline). The three-letter abbreviations beneath the full names are used in other figures and in the text.

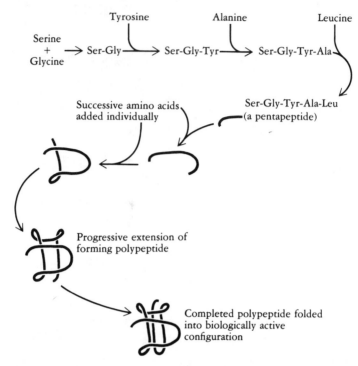

FIGURE 2 Amino acids are assembled into chainlike polymers called polypeptides. The three-dimensional configuration of a completed polypeptide is uniquely established by its sequence of amino acids and by the ways individual amino acids interact with one another and with the fluid surrounding the polypeptide. The three-dimensional configuration, in turn, determines biological functions and activities.

cleotide strand to which the organic bases of the nucleotide subunits are attached (Figure 3).

It is the sequence of organic bases along the sugar–phosphate backbone that contains the genetic information in a polynucleotide. A portion of an imaginary DNA might accordingly be abbreviated as

. . .-A-C-C-A-T-C-T-A-G-C-T-G-G-. . .

DNA molecules as they usually occur in cells consist of two

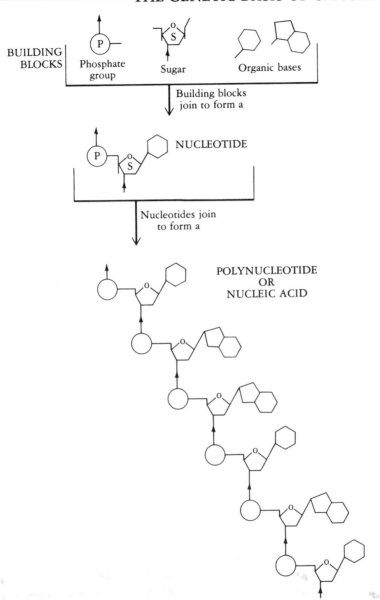

FIGURE 3   General structure of nucleic acid polymers.

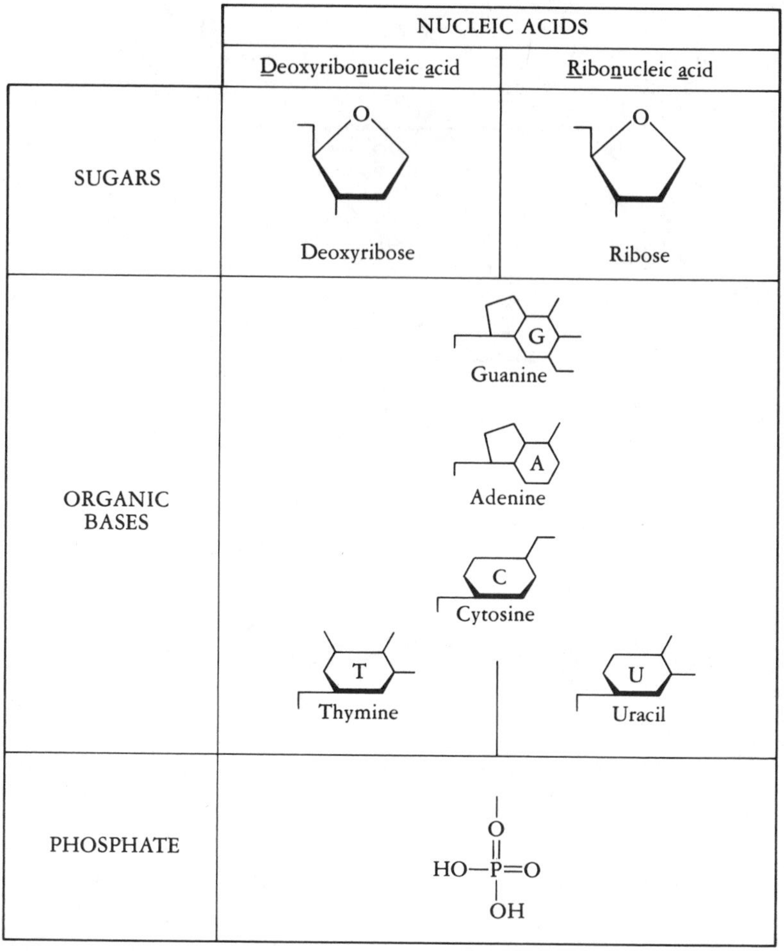

NUCLEIC ACIDS		
	Deoxyribonucleic acid	Ribonucleic acid
SUGARS	Deoxyribose	Ribose
ORGANIC BASES		
	Guanine	
	Adenine	
	Cytosine	
	Thymine	Uracil
PHOSPHATE	$HO-P=O$ with O double-bonded above and OH below	

FIGURE 4   The building blocks of DNAs and RNAs.

strands that come together to form a ladder-like macromolecule (Figure 5). The series of sugar–phosphate groups correspond to the sides of the ladder; pairs of nucleotides correspond to the rungs. In a given segment of double-stranded DNA, the sequence of nucleotides in one strand determines precisely the sequence of nucleotides in the other strand. This is a result of the ways in which the organic bases interact with one another.

Base A has a shape that matches well with the shape of base T. Similarly, base G matches base C. A-T pairs and C-G pairs are called COMPLEMENTARY BASE PAIRS. The two bases in each complementary pair (AT, TA, GC, and CG) attract each other weakly (dashed lines in Figure 5). Two strands of complementary base pairs are called COMPLEMENTARY STRANDS. Together, weak chemical attractions between many thousands of complementary base pairs add up to an attraction strong

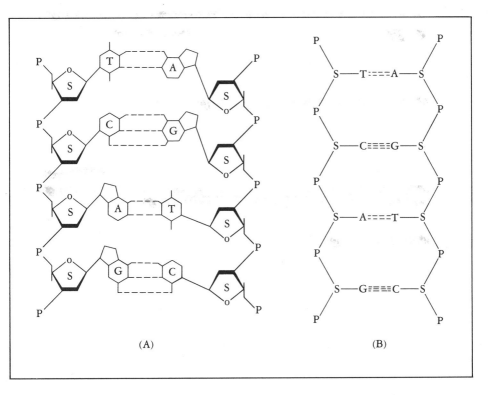

(A)   (B)

FIGURE 5   Two representations of a segment of double-stranded DNA held together by hydrogen bonds (dashed lines) between complementary base pairs. Part (A) shows more details of the orientation of deoxyribose sugars, S, and organic bases A, T, G, and C; in (B) each component is abbreviated by a single letter. Note that A and T form hydrogen bonds, as do G and C.

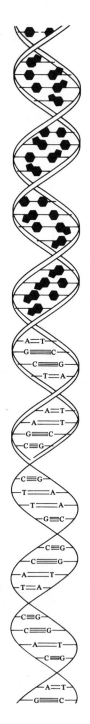

enough to hold two complementary strands together to form a stable, ladder-like molecule. Thus, a segment of two-stranded DNA containing the imaginary strand listed earlier might be represented as

...-A-C-C-A-T-C-T-A-G-C-T-G-G-...
...-T-G-G-T-A-G-A-T-C-G-A-C-C-...

However, the two complementary strands of native DNA are not simply parallel in the same way as the rails of a ladder. The organic bases are attached to the sugar–phosphate backbones so that each nucleotide pair is rotated slightly with respect to the pairs above and below it, rather like the treads in a spiral staircase. For this reason, complementary polynucleotide strands twist around each other to form what is called a double helix, or a duplex molecule (Figure 6). The genetic information carried in a human chromosome is coded in a DNA duplex that is on the average about 3 cm (just under 1.25 inches) long and that consists of millions of complementary nucleotide pairs arranged in a linear sequence. Each protein that a cell can make is coded by a specific segment of a DNA duplex; that segment is called a GENE. Thus, the long DNA duplex molecule in a human chromosome is, in effect, a string of genes.

At the end of each cell cycle, each of the two daughter cells receives identical copies of all chromosomes; hence each receives a full set of parental genes.

The DNA duplex in each chromosome must have duplicated earlier in that cycle to yield two identical copies. Without high-fidelity duplication, a cell's descendants could not long survive. The complementarity of the polynucleotide chains in

FIGURE 6 Complementary polynucleotide strands intertwine to form double-stranded DNA molecules with characteristic helical shapes. Here, the sugar–phosphate backbone is represented by two ribbons, the complementary bases by silhouettes (above) and by one-letter abbreviations (below).

the DNA duplex is the basis for the required high-fidelity replication.

As replication of a DNA duplex begins, the two complementary strands unwind and separate from one another as shown in Figure 7A. Newly produced individual nucleotides match up with nucleotides in the template chains according to the base-pairing rules like those that function to hold the DNA duplex together: A with T, T with A, C with G, and G with C (Figure 7B). As the individual nucleotides match up to the templates, they themselves are joined into a new polynucleotide chain (Figure 7C) in a reaction catalyzed by the enzyme DNA polymerase. Thus a new, exactly complementary strand forms along *each* of the two separated parental strands (Figure 7D). Each new chain and its template wind about each other as the new chain grows, automatically forming a new DNA duplex. When the process is completed, two complete double helices are formed, identical in nucleotide sequence to one another *and* to the parental duplex. It is worth noting that one strand of each new duplex is in fact *the same strand* that was in the parental duplex: only two new strands are formed at each replication.

DNA Genes Act Through RNA Messages

The discussion to this point has considered two classes of cellular macromolecules: DNAs and the proteins they specify. Attention now shifts to a third important class of macromolecules: the ribonucleic acids (RNAs), which are an essential link between genes and proteins.

Like DNA, a molecule of RNA is a polymer of nucleotides arranged in a linear sequence. Each nucleotide in an RNA consists of a sugar molecule, a phosphate group, and an organic base, just as in DNA. There are, however, important differences between the sugars and bases of RNAs and those of DNA (Figure 4). First, instead of deoxyribose, RNA nucleotides contain the slightly different sugar ribose. Second, instead of the organic base thymine (T), RNAs contain the slightly

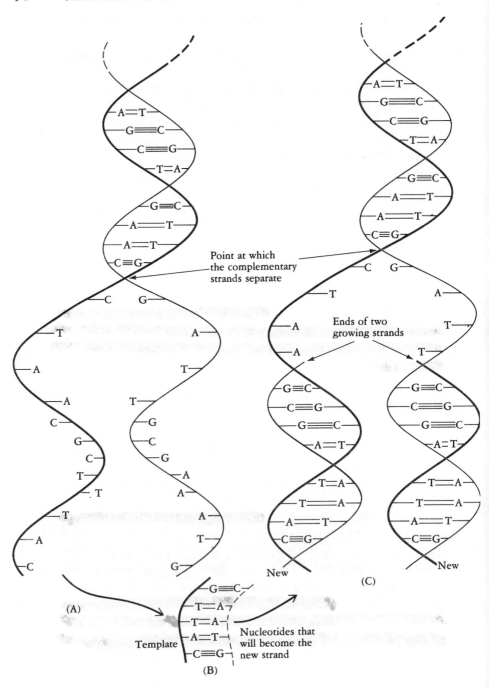

Point at which
the complementary
strands separate

Ends of two
growing strands

(A)

Template

New

(C)

New

G≡C
T=A
T=A
A=T
C≡G

Nucleotides that
will become the
new strand

(B)

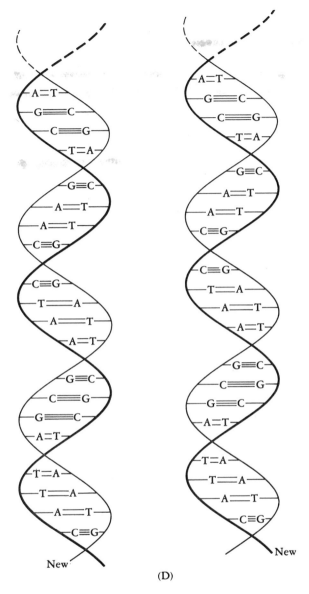

(D)

FIGURE 7 Replication of part of a DNA duplex. (A) Complementary strands separate, exposing unpaired nucleotides. (B) Nucleotides that will become a new strand become paired (by hydrogen bonding) with nucleotides on the existing (template) strand. (C) Chemical bonds join adjacent nucleotides into new strands exactly complementary to each strand of the duplex being replicated. (D) The two identical duplexes formed from the original duplex in (A). Each consists of one strand from the original duplex and a newly synthesized, complementary strand.

different organic base uracil (U); the bases A, G, and C occur in the nucleotides of both RNAs and DNAs, as does the phosphate group. One consequence of these differences is that native DNAs usually form double helices, whereas RNA chains do not.

All RNAs are formed in the nucleus but function in the cytoplasm and must move out through the nuclear membrane. An important class of RNA known as messenger RNA (mRNA) carries information from the genes to the protein-making machinery in the cytoplasm (Figure 8).

When a gene is active, the two chains of its DNA duplex separate. One of the chains then acts as a template for the

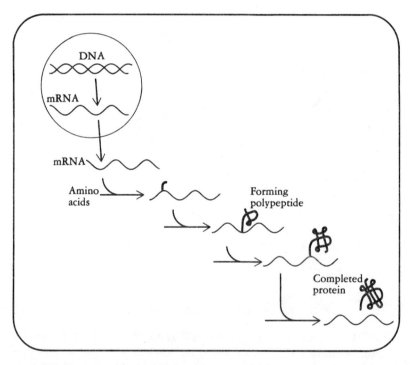

FIGURE 8 Messenger RNA molecules (mRNA) made in the nucleus are copies of DNA genes. The mRNA molecules are transferred to the cytoplasm, where they guide the joining of amino acids into polypeptide chains. The polypeptide chain folds up (Figure 2) to form the final protein product.

formation of an mRNA molecule (Figure 9). The mRNA is assembled according to base-pairing rules that are similar to those that govern the replication of DNAs. Wherever the DNA template contains a G, C, or T nucleotide, it is paired with a C, G, or A nucleotide, respectively, just as in the replication of DNA. And, as in the replication of DNA, the matched nucleotides are linked together into a polynucleotide chain by an enzyme, RNA polymerase in this case. Wherever the DNA template contains an A nucleotide, however, it becomes paired with a U nucleotide that is then incorporated into the forming RNA copy by the RNA polymerase.

This entire process, which is completed in only a few minutes, yields an mRNA polynucleotide that contains the same number of nucleotides as the DNA template (gene) on which it was formed. The nucleotides in the mRNA polynucleotide occur in a linear sequence precisely specified by the DNA template. The new mRNA polynucleotide then separates from its template, enabling the entire process to be repeated many times. This results in many identical mRNA copies of the same stretch of DNA. This process of copying the information in part of a DNA molecule (a gene) into an mRNA molecule is called the TRANSCRIPTION of a DNA gene into RNA.

The mRNA molecules carry genetic messages from genes in the nucleus to the protein-forming machinery in the cytoplasm. The main elements of the protein-forming machinery are the cytoplasmic particles called ribosomes. The mRNA molecules bind to ribosomes, and with the help of the ribosomes, the mRNAs are used to direct the synthesis of protein molecules. In this process each mRNA molecule may be used over and over. In this way, many identical protein molecules may be produced from a single mRNA molecule that is acting as a template. Thus, as genetic information flows from nucleus to cytoplasm, it can be amplified at two points: many copies of a messenger RNA can be made from a single DNA template, and in turn, many protein molecules can be made under the guidance of each RNA message (Figure 9). The RNA-guided assembly of amino acid chains to form proteins is called TRANSLATION.

RNA messages do have limited life spans. After guiding

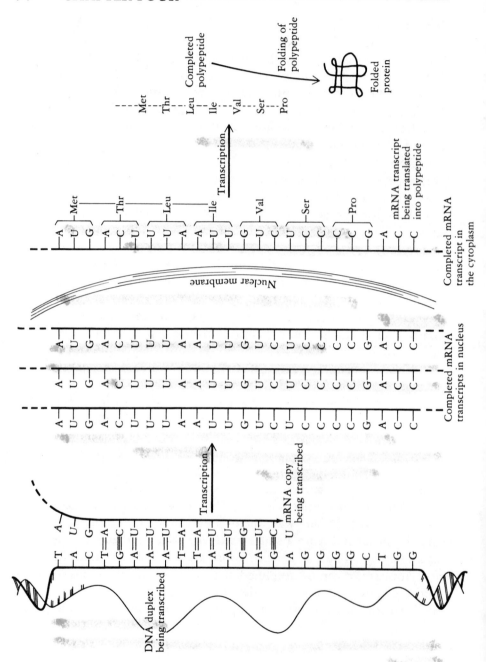

◀ FIGURE 9   DNA specifies the sequence of amino acids in a polypeptide. (A) Part of a DNA duplex unwinds and serves as a template for
the transcription of a complementary strand of mRNA. (B) Many
mRNA transcripts may be made of a segment of DNA, and all pass
through the nuclear membrane into the cytoplasm. (C) In the cytoplasm,
each mRNA transcript is translated into a polypeptide as amino acids
are linked together in the sequence specified by the mRNA. Each
transcript may be translated several or many times before being destroyed. (D) The forming polypeptide automatically folds into a unique
three-dimensional shape determined by the sequence of its amino acids.

the synthesis of some number of copies of a particular kind of
protein molecule, the RNA template is destroyed by the cell.
The manner in which cells regulate the life spans of different
mRNAs is not known, but an important consequence of this
regulation is that the continuous synthesis of a given type of
protein requires the continuous production of the appropriate
mRNA messages. If the synthesis of the RNA message is
stopped, the production of the particular protein in turn will
stop, usually in a matter of hours. By regulating the synthesis
of various kinds of mRNAs, a cell controls the kinds of proteins
it synthesizes at a given time.

To recapitulate: the sequence of nucleotides in a DNA
gene dictates the sequence of nucleotides in an RNA message;
the RNA message moves to the cytoplasm and there dictates
the sequence of amino acids in a protein molecule; the sequence of amino acids in the protein, in turn, determines the
unique physical and chemical properties of that kind of macromolecule and thus the properties and behavior of the cell in
which all this occurs. In short, DNA codes for RNA, which
codes for protein, which determines what a cell is like. The
following sketch encapsulates this flow of genetic information
as described so far.

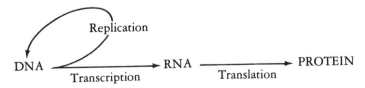

It is worth remembering that all three arrows in this sketch represent sequences of reactions catalyzed by enzymes; enzymes are themselves proteins that are generated by the same flow of information.

Transcription and Translation Involve a Universal Genetic Code

It remains only to explain the way information for making proteins is coded into sequences of nucleotides in DNA and RNA. The four kinds of nucleotides in DNA molecules correspond to the four letters in a GENETIC CODE. Each gene is a linear sequence of many hundreds of these four nucleotide letters. What gives each of the thousands of genes in a human cell its unique quality, its meaning, is the linear sequence in which the four nucleotides are arranged in that gene. The letters of a human language alphabet are used analogously: what gives an array of letters its meaning is the linear sequence of those letters and the spacers between them. So it is with the genetic code.

Transcription of DNA into RNA converts one four-letter code consisting of G, C, A, and T into another four-letter code consisting instead of G, C, A, and U. The base-pairing rules built into the code assure that a given nucleotide sequence in DNA will be faithfully transcribed into an equivalent sequence in the RNA made from it. A DNA polynucleotide such as

$$\ldots\text{-T-C-A-G-A-T-C-A-G-T-G-G-}\ldots$$

is thus uniquely transcribed into the corresponding RNA polynucleotide

$$\ldots\text{-A-G-U-C-U-A-G-U-C-A-C-C-}\ldots$$

Because the RNA code involves only the letters G, C, A, and U and because there are 20 different amino acids to be encoded, a single RNA nucleotide cannot encode an amino acid—there are 16 too few RNA letters. A simple alternative is an RNA code that uses a *pair* of successive letters to specify a single amino acid word: AU might code for one amino acid, UA for another, CA for another, AC for another, and so on. But this generates only 16 different combinations (AA, AU, AG, AC; UA, UU, UG, UC; GA, GU, GG, GC; CA, CU, CG, CC), still four short of the number needed to encode 20 amino acids. A code with three letters per word would yield 64 different combinations, 44 *more* words than the 20 that seem to be needed. Four letters per word should yield 256 words, and so forth.

A number of ingenious experiments have proved that the RNA code involves "words" made up of *three* consecutive nucleotides: it is a TRIPLET CODE. For example, the triplet of letters CUA in RNA encodes the amino acid leucine; GUU prescribes the amino acid valine. The 64 different triplets that can be made from a four-letter code are more than three times as many as the 20 amino acids to be encoded. Several different triplets code for the same amino acid. Table 1 lists the amino acid coded by each of the 64 triplets. Note that six different triplets all designate the amino acid leucine, and six designate arginine. By contrast, only one triplet designates methionine, and only one triplet designates the amino acid tryptophan. Other amino acids are designated by two to five triplets. Because in several cases a given amino acid is specified by more than one triplet, the code is termed DEGENERATE. The origin and significance of this redundancy is not understood. Three triplets (UAA, UAG, and UGA) are used to designate the end of the message and are analogous to the period at the end of a sentence. Where one gene ends and the next one begins is marked in the DNA molecule by certain sequences of bases. For example, the end of a gene may be a long stretch consisting only of AT base pairs. The beginning of a gene is also a form of punctuation along the DNA molecule and consists of a particular sequence of nucleotides, but this sequence is complicated and not yet well understood.

The manner in which a protein can be uniquely specified

TABLE 1. The triplet RNA code. To determine the triplet code(s) for an amino acid, read across the table for the first two nucleotides; the third nucleotide is at the head of the column in which the amino acid is listed. For example, phenylalanine (Phe) is coded by two triplets, UUU and UUC. The triplets UAA, UAG, and UGA signal the end of a gene and function as *stop* signals.

First Nucleotide	Second Nucleotide	Third Nucleotide			
		U	C	A	G
U	U	Phe	Phe	Leu	Leu
U	C	Ser	Ser	Ser	Ser
U	A	Tyr	Tyr	END	END
U	G	Cys	Cys	END	Trp
C	U	Leu	Leu	Leu	Leu
C	C	Pro	Pro	Pro	Pro
C	A	His	His	Gln	Gln
C	G	Arg	Arg	Arg	Arg
A	U	Ile	Ile	Ile	Met
A	C	Thr	Thr	Thr	Thr
A	A	Asn	Asn	Lys	Lys
A	G	Ser	Ser	Arg	Arg
G	U	Val	Val	Val	Val
G	C	Ala	Ala	Ala	Ala
G	A	Asp	Asp	Glu	Glu
G	G	Gly	Gly	Gly	Gly

by a length of DNA or RNA can now be summarized:

```
...┼T-C-A┼G-A-T┼C-A-G┼T-G-G┼...    DNA
                                    ↓ ←── transcription
...┼A-G-U┼C-U-A┼G-U-C┼A-C-C┼...    RNA
                                    ↓ ←── translation
...┼- Ser -┼- Leu -┼- Val -┼- Thr -┼...   PROTEIN
```

In this way, a gene is not merely a piece of a chromosome but more precisely a sequence of deoxyribonucleotides that encode a single protein (summarized in Figure 9). In the economy of the cell, the transfer of information from a gene into protein molecules may be visualized diagrammatically as in Figure 10.

The genetic code is universal in the sense that all life forms known, from bacteria to humans, employ exactly the same genetic code in the same way. Indeed, proteins can be synthesized in test tubes by mixing DNA from one organism with RNA polymerase from another species and ribosomes from a third, along with an appropriate supply of small building blocks and a source of energy. This universality of the genetic code permits application of information and insights gained through the study of nonhuman organisms (including bacteria and viruses) to the study of human cells. Although such inferences

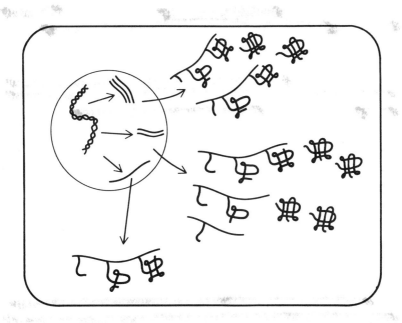

FIGURE 10   The flow of genetic information from DNA to proteins. Many messenger RNAs are transcribed from each DNA gene. These mRNAs move from the nucleus into the cytoplasm, where they are translated into proteins. Each mRNA molecule can direct the assembly of many identical protein molecules.

across species and kingdoms of organisms are not without some risk, they are often extremely useful, as discussed in later chapters.

Transcription of DNA into RNA involves many enzymes other than RNA polymerase, the only one mentioned thus far. Translation of mRNA into protein similarly involves many enzymes not mentioned here, as well as the participation of many proteins and ribosomes.

Mutations Result from Alterations in DNA

DNA can be damaged in several ways, most of which lead to genetic damage (MUTATIONS). Seen at the molecular level, a mutation is an alteration in a number or sequence of nucleotide pairs in part of a cell's DNA.

Agents such as ionizing radiations, as well as some chemical mutagens, can induce physical breaks in DNA duplexes. Most cells make enzymes that repair such breaks, but these repair enzymes are not perfectly efficient, and such repairs are not invariably exact. A small fragment of DNA, even a fragment as small as a single nucleotide pair, may be left out during the repair. Such a small DELETION is a gene mutation that may have profound effects. Every DNA molecule replicated against a DNA template carrying a deletion also will carry the deletion. Every RNA message transcribed from such a mutated gene will be translated into a chain of amino acids with a sequence that is abnormal from the site of the deletion to the end of the amino acid chain (Figure 11). The significance to the cell of a deletion mutation depends on the size and location of the deletion within a gene, on the resulting change in the protein coded by the mutated gene, and on the importance of that protein in the cell's economy.

Deletions of one or a few nucleotide pairs are called FRAME-SHIFT MUTATIONS because of the way in which they alter the translation of RNA triplets. Some deletions involve losses of so much DNA (so many genes) that the structure of the mutated chromosome is detectably altered. Needless to say, deletions of any size may produce profound changes in the affected gene, generally by eliminating the normal protein and its role in the cell.

Another class of mutations that are caused by some kinds of chemical mutagens consists of the substitution of one nucleotide pair in place of another, for example, changing an AT pair to a GC pair (Figure 12). Such a POINT MUTATION may alter the information carried by a triplet so that a different amino acid is inserted in the protein coded by the mutated gene. Although a gene may consist of hundreds of nucleotide pairs, changing only one pair (and thus changing only one amino acid out of several hundred amino acids) may be sufficient to impair severely the function of the protein coded by that gene.

An example of such a point mutation occurs in the case of the protein hemoglobin. Hemoglobin is the major protein of red blood cells and is responsible for the red color of blood. This protein binds to oxygen in the lungs and carries it to various cells, where the oxygen is released. Hemoglobin contains two different amino acid chains: the α and β chains. The β chain is made up of 146 amino acids that begin with the sequence

```
 1    2    3    4    5    6    7    8
Val - His - Leu - Thr - Pro - Glu - Glu - Lys - . . . - . . . -
```

The genetic disease known as sickle cell anemia is the result of a point mutation in the gene that codes for the β chain. The point mutation causes valine rather than the normal glutamic acid to be inserted in the sixth position of β chains.

mutant β chain

```
 1    2    3    4    5    6    7    8
Val - His - Leu - Thr - Pro - VAL - Glu - Lys - . . . - . . . -
```

The substitution of this one amino acid drastically alters the ability of the β chain to function properly. Therefore, the

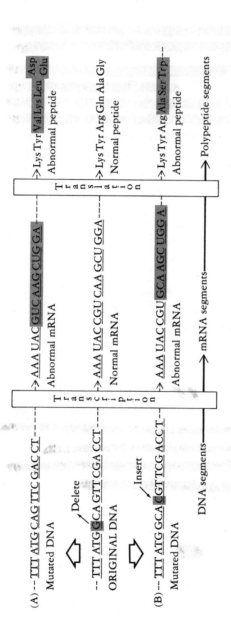

FIGURE 11 Frameshift mutations result when one or more nucleotides are (A) deleted from or (B) inserted into a segment of DNA. Because nucleic acids are decoded in clusters of three nucleotides (triplet codons), deletions and insertions may change the makeup of all triplets beyond the site of the mutation. DNAs that sustain frameshift mutations are transcribed into abnormal mRNAs, which code for abnormal polypeptides. Depending on where in a gene such frameshift mutations occur and on their number, the abnormal polypeptides may function normally, abnormally, or not at all.

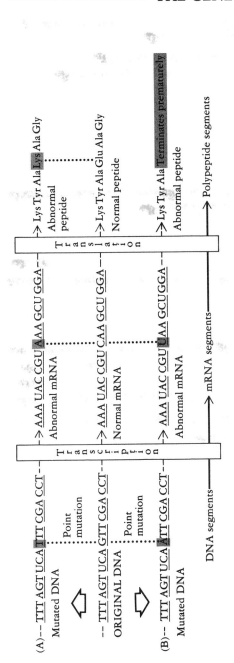

FIGURE 12   Two possible consequences of point mutations. In (A), a point mutation converts GTT to TTT. The mutated DNA is transcribed into an mRNA in which CAA is replaced by AAA. This message codes for an abnormal polypeptide in which glutamine is replaced by lysine. In (B), the mutated DNA (GTT to ATT) is transcribed into an mRNA that contains a "stop" signal (the codon UAA) in an inappropriate position. This signal prematurely terminates the translation of abnormal mRNA, resulting in a truncated polypeptide. Depending on where in a gene such point mutations occur, the abnormal polypeptides may function normally, abnormally, or not at all.

hemoglobin molecules fail to transport oxygen normally, leading to the condition of sickle cell anemia.

Point mutations may also occur spontaneously. The replication of DNA involves the enzyme DNA polymerase, which catalyzes the joining of nucleotides into a new DNA duplex. By means not fully understood this enzyme ordinarily adds only nucleotides that are complementary to the template chain. Extremely rarely, however, a mispairing occurs and the enzyme inserts an incorrect nucleotide. For example, it may allow the incorrect pairing of a C with a T or with an A. Even more rarely, these mispairings are stabilized and persist as alterations in the nucleotide sequence, as mutations. This kind of spontaneous error occurs at most about once for every 10 billion nucleotides added. Such errors, which may be due to thermal "noise," are, nevertheless, inherited as point mutations. Most mutations, however, are the result of the mutagenic action on DNA of certain chemicals (Chapter 7) or radiation (Chapter 8).

Thus, a mutation in a gene may cause a defect in or complete loss of a protein needed for one or another cell function. In many cases this leads to death of the cell, in which case the change in the gene is known as a LETHAL MUTATION. Mutations are extraordinarily important in causing cancer. Mutation of genes that code for proteins essential for the regulation of cell reproduction and differentiation is almost certainly the basis of most human cancer. It is in this important sense that cancer is an inherited disease at the cellular level. After this brief description of molecular genetics and mutation, attention now shifts to a discussion of cancer and heredity.

5

Cancer and Heredity

THE preceding chapter described the molecular basis of inheritance, including the nature of mutations and how they are transmitted from a cell to its progeny. Cancer was characterized as a result of mutations that remove controls that normally act in the G1 period of the cell cycle. Cells with such mutations continue to divide when their normal counterparts do not, and they do not differentiate when their normal counterparts do.[1] In this chapter, we turn to whole organisms and examine how cancer is inherited from generation to generation.

It is well documented that many kinds of human cancers tend to occur more often in some families than in others. Many family histories provide evidence that a *tendency* to develop a certain kind of cancer can be inherited, that is, passed on from parent to offspring. In some cases, this inherited tendency to develop cancer is strong. Many, although not all, members of a family will develop a particular form of cancer. Such "cancer families" are rare but are unmistakable when they do occur. In other cases, the inherited tendency may be so slight as to be barely detectable. So few members of stricken families develop a particular cancer that the tendency is recognized only when the experiences of many families are combined.

Although a tendency to develop some kinds of cancer is

clearly inherited, heredity is certainly not implicated in all kinds of cancers. The fact that a family has no history of a hereditary form of cancer by no means guarantees that all members of the family will continue to escape that cancer. Nor does even a strong family history of some form of cancer doom any particular member of the family to the disease.

Our understanding of how a tendency to develop cancer passes from generation to generation is still very incomplete. A tendency for humans to develop cancer can be inherited directly through the genes, but only a few such examples are known. Although inheritance through the genes is likely in most cases, there are other ways a tendency to develop cancer might cross generations. There is, for example, the experimental evidence that cancer-causing viruses are transmitted from parent to offspring among mice (see Chapter 9). Indeed, much of what is known about inherited tendencies to develop cancer comes from studies with laboratory animals.

Susceptibility to Some Cancers Is Inherited in Laboratory Animals

Many difficulties of investigating the inheritance of cancer in humans are avoided by studying laboratory animals whose breeding can be manipulated and controlled. Inbred strains of mice are particularly useful. In contrast to the 25-year generation time in humans, the generation time in mice is a matter of a few months. The life span of humans is about 70 years, that of mice about 2 years. And of course, the matings required in genetic studies are easy to arrange and control in laboratory mice. In addition, controlling exposures to cancer-causing agents such as radiation, viruses, cigarette smoke, and various chemicals is clearly easier with laboratory animals than with humans.

Studies with animals are not foolproof, however. In 1979, cancer researchers were distressed to learn that at least one of the standard laboratory diets for rodents was contaminated with significant amounts of powerful chemical carcinogens known as nitrosamines (see Chapter 7).[2] Contaminated food could easily distort laboratory experiments about preventing, inducing, and treating cancer. Such technical difficulties are usually recognized and eliminated in a timely way. More fundamental are the biochemical and physiological differences that make rodents and other laboratory animals only approximate models for humans. These differences are well known to cancer researchers and usually restrain uncritical extrapolation from animals to humans. Properly performed and interpreted, animal studies provide important insights into what cancer is and how to deal with it. The following examples illustrate the kinds of insights about cancer that have come from studies of laboratory animals of many kinds.

BREAST CANCER AND LEUKEMIA IN MICE

Researchers can use selective breeding programs to produce strains of laboratory animals, particularly mice and rats, that are either very resistant or very susceptible to certain cancers. For example, certain inbred strains of mice are extremely susceptible to leukemia, and most of the animals ultimately develop this form of cancer. Some inbred mouse strains develop breast cancer at extremely high rates; other inbred strains develop breast cancer very rarely. In the particular cases of leukemia and breast cancer in mice, what is inherited seems to be a SUSCEPTIBILITY to cancer. In both cases, the cancers are *caused* by viruses, but a *susceptibility* to the viruses is inherited (Chapter 9).[3] Breast cancer and leukemia (and many other kinds of cancers) can also be induced in mice by radiation (Chapter 8) or chemical carcinogens (Chapter 7). The extent to which susceptibility to these agents is inherited is still an important but poorly understood problem.

MELANOMA IN TROPICAL FISH

One of the first and still best understood demonstrations of directly inherited cancer comes from studies of a tropical fish known as the *platy*. The cancer is a melanoma, a common form of cancer that results from the uncontrolled proliferation of pigment-containing cells, usually in the skin. The pigment cells that are affected in the platy are black and occur in the fish's dorsal fin (Figure 1A). Melanomas never develop in normal platys or in a closely related species known as *swordtails,* which lack black pigment cells in their dorsal fins. When a platy is mated with a swordtail, some of the hybrid offspring are fertile and generally normal but may have pigment cells in their dorsal fins. These pigment cells tend to divide somewhat more often in the hybrids, becoming more numerous than in the pure platy (Figure 1B). If a platy × swordtail *hybrid* is mated with a swordtail, some of the offspring of this mating again have pigmented cells in their dorsal fins. Now, however, the dorsal pigment cells reproduce so much more rapidly that large malignant tumors form in many of the hybrids. The tumors spread throughout the body of a hybrid fish, eventually killing it (Figure 1C).

Genetic analyses provide the following explanation of how these melanomas are inherited.[4] In purebred platys, the reproduction of the pigment cells in the dorsal fin is strictly controlled by a number of regulatory genes that are always present. Purebred swordtails, which have no pigment cells in their dorsal fins, reasonably enough have no such regulatory genes— they would be superfluous in the swordtail. A platy × swordtail hybrid has on the average half the normal platy's complement of these regulatory genes. Pigment cells in the dorsal fin of these hybrids therefore reproduce slightly more often than in the pure platy (Figure 1B). When a hybrid is crossed with a swordtail, the number of regulatory genes in their offspring is further reduced. As a result, the pigment cells are now so poorly controlled that they proliferate rapidly, forming tumors that kill the fish.

Melanoma in platy × swordtail hybrids is one of the best understood cases of how cancer is inherited and is an important precedent for developing ideas about how other animals, including humans, might inherit cancer.

BRAIN CANCER IN THE FRUIT FLY

Another clear case of an inherited cancer involves the common fruit fly. The fruit fly is in many ways uniquely suited for genetic experimentation, and much of what is known about

(A)

(B)

(C)

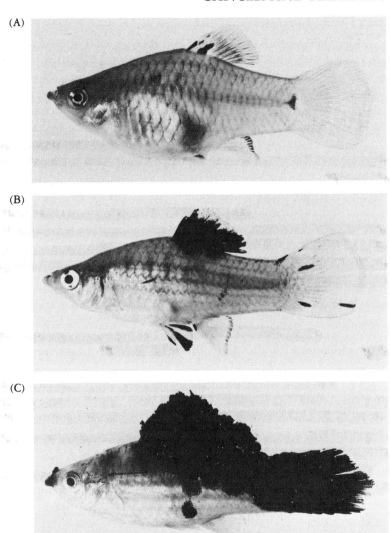

FIGURE 1   Melanoma in hybrids of platy fish and swordtails. (A) A normal platy fish with two spots in its dorsal fin that contain pigmented cells. (B) A *platy* × *swordtail* hybrid has many more pigmented cells in its dorsal fin. (C) Offspring of a mating between a hybrid and a swordtail has even more pigmented cells, in its dorsal fin and elsewhere. Control over the reproduction of these pigmented cells is defective, and these fish are eventually killed by the resulting melanomas.[4]

heredity was first developed through studies of the fruit fly.

The type of cancer in question was discovered accidentally in a laboratory colony of fruit flies. The cancer forms during the larval (caterpillar) state of the fly's development, always in cells that normally become the brain cells responsible for vision in the adult. These future brain cells proliferate excessively, fail to differentiate normally, and kill the fly before it matures.

Genetic analyses established that this cancer is inherited through a single gene, apparently a mutated form of a regulatory gene. When male and female flies, each carrying the mutated gene, are mated, the cancer occurs in about one-fourth of all their offspring.[5] It appears that the normal version of the relevant gene is required to regulate the reproduction of the brain cells during development. The mutated form of the gene fails to exert the normal degree of control, permitting the growth of abnormal cells that produce a cancer.

These and similar studies of inherited cancer in animals show that cancer can begin when crucial regulatory genes are lost (melanoma in the platy fish) or mutated (brain tumor in the fruit fly). Such examples are important for at least two reasons. First, continued analyses of cases like these may yield new, fundamental understandings of the molecular mechanisms that regulate the reproduction of cells. Second, these findings require serious consideration of the possibility that cancer-causing chemicals, radiation, and viruses (see Chapters 6 through 9) may actually cause cancer by causing mutations or malfunctions of regulatory genes. On the basis of this, inherited tendencies to develop cancers in humans will be considered in the next section.

Some Human Cancers Run in Families

As mentioned earlier, some common human cancers cluster in families: relatives of cancer patients develop the same kind of cancer far more often than expected from the frequency of that cancer in the general population. Familial tendencies are known for cancers of the breast, stomach, colon, uterus, prostate, and lung and for some leukemias. For some cancers, particularly childhood cancers and cancers of the breast or colon, the rate among blood relatives can be as much as 20 to 30 times higher than among nonrelatives.[6] Such higher rates of particular cancers within families are strong evidence of hereditary predispositions to develop those cancers.

In addition to overly frequent cancers of the same kind within a family, it occasionally happens that many members of the same family will develop different kinds of cancers. For example, in one family of five, the mother developed cancers in both breasts at the age of 32, one son had bone cancer at the age of 15, the other son developed a cartilage cancer at age 22, and the only daughter developed a brain tumor at 19. Four of the five members of this family had highly malignant cancers at unusually young ages.[6] Fortunately, such cancer families are rare. Because on the average, cancer afflicts one person out of four in the United States, it is reasonable to expect about one cancer in this family.[7] More significant is the early onset of cancers in this family. One would have expected no cancer to occur in this family because the rate of cancer among people younger than 40 is far less than one in four. *Any* cancer in this family is thus surprising; so many cancers at such early ages is most unusual. However, it is often the case with familial cancer that the cancers begin at early ages, often in childhood, for example, leukemias, neuroblastoma (nerve cell cancer), and certain kidney cancers.

Even when a very strong tendency to inherit a familial cancer is clear, an individual may never develop the particular cancer. A number of careful studies of some human cancers and many animal cancers indicate, in fact, that familial cancers almost always reflect the inheritance of a *predisposition* to cancer.[8] The individual who is hereditarily predisposed to develop cancer probably develops the disease only as a result of exposure to cancer-causing environmental agent(s). These environmental agents are probably almost always cancer-causing chemicals, radiation, or certain kinds of viruses. In other words, an inherited predisposition to cancer is not enough to provoke the disease. The individual must also be exposed to some agent that brings out the susceptibility. It is as if the body's normal defenses against cancer are less effective in persons who are genetically predisposed to the disease. Although a complete understanding of how heredity affects the chance an individual will develop this or that kind of cancer remains far off, clear evidence that heredity plays a role in the development of a few human cancers is in hand. Some examples follow.

CANCER OF THE EYE: RETINOBLASTOMA

RETINOBLASTOMA is a rare cancer of the eye and occurs in about 1 child in 18,000, usually before the age of 3. A human eye contains many millions of retinal cells, and a child afflicted with retinoblastoma may develop several tumors, each arising from a single retinal cell—the average number of tumors is three. The tumors may all occur in one eye (unilateral retinoblastoma) or be distributed between both eyes (bilateral retinoblastoma).[9] Tumors do not form once the child has reached the age of 4 or 5, probably because all retinal cells, which are really nerve cells, have differentiated to the point of permanent arrest in the G1 period of the cell cycle. Cells that have stopped dividing, as discussed in Chapter 2, can no longer be converted into cancer cells.

The retinoblastoma tumor, if untreated, grows inward from the eye along the optic nerve to the brain. Tumor cells may also metastasize through the blood to the liver, spleen, kidneys, or bones. In either event, before modern methods of treatment retinoblastoma was usually fatal at an early age, and few victims reached the age of reproduction. This minimized the hereditary spread of the disease. Retinoblastoma victims can now often be cured by surgery (removal of the affected eye) or by radiation treatment and chemotherapy. Many victims now live to reproduce, with consequences described below.

Retinoblastoma occurs in both hereditary and nonhereditary forms, and new cases of the hereditary type arise constantly. Only about 10 percent of retinoblastoma victims have a familial history of the disease. These persons inherit not the actual disease but a high susceptibility to the disease—a susceptibility that may or may not be activated. Persons who inherit a susceptibility can pass it on to their children. Of the 90 percent who have no prior familial history of retinoblastoma, about half can transmit the disease to their children.

A simple two-part hypothesis accounts for these patterns in the ways retinoblastoma strikes. Assume that young retinal cells develop under the control of a particular regulatory gene. Assume also that only one of the two copies of this gene present in each retinal cell needs to function in order for development to be normal.[10] There are ample data to support each assumption. The following three possibilities exist. (1) Inheriting two defective copies of the regulatory gene, one from each parent, would presumably cause all retinal cells to become cancerous, probably early in fetal development, most likely with fatal consequences. No instance of such a live birth is known and would escape detection in aborted fetuses. (2) Persons who inherit one defective copy and one functional copy of the regulatory gene will be susceptible to the disease. They would develop retinoblastoma tumors each time a young retinal cell sustained a mutation that inactivated its single functional copy of the regulatory gene. Such susceptible persons who survive to reproduce will pass on a similar susceptibility to about half the offspring they produce with a normal mate. (3) Persons who inherit two functional copies of the regulatory gene would ordinarily escape the disease. *Both* copies of the regulatory gene in a *single* retinal cell would have to be mutated during the first few years of life in order for a normal person to develop retinoblastoma. This is a most unlikely coincidence of rare events, as demonstrated by the rarity of the disease in the general population. Moreover, such individuals would not pass susceptibility to their children because the mutations were not in germ cells.[11] These circumstances would account for rare instances of retinoblastoma among persons without family histories of the disease in prior or subsequent generations.

According to this hypothesis, then, inheriting susceptibility to retinoblastoma results from inheriting one mutated copy of a regulatory gene so that a subsequent mutation to the other copy can convert a normal retinal cell into one in which G1 arrest is abnormal. This hypothesis, which explains how susceptibility to retinoblastoma can be inherited when there is a familial history of the disease, also explains how new cases of hereditary retinoblastoma can arise. The explanation again calls for two mutations, but to different cells. Suppose that the first mutation, the one that establishes susceptibility, occurs in a germ cell of a normal individual. He or she will not be susceptible to retinoblastoma because the mutation does not affect any retinal cells. If a germ cell with the mutated regulatory gene happens to form a new individual, all the cells of that new individual—including all germ cells and all retinal cells—will carry the first mutation. This person will be susceptible to retinoblastoma, that is, susceptible to the effect of a second, environmentally induced mutation to a retinal cell. This person also will be able to pass the first mutation on to his or her children. New hereditary lines of retinoblastoma might well originate in this way.

FAMILIAL BREAST CANCER

About 1 in 12 American women develops breast cancer during her lifetime—one of the highest rates in the world for this cancer. The rate increased slightly from 1920 to 1970 but has remained essentially constant for at least the last 10 years. In Japan, by contrast, only about 1 woman in 60 develops breast cancer. This rate has also increased over the last 20 years, by about 50 percent, particularly in large cities, and it continues to rise.[12]

The cause(s) of breast cancer remain poorly understood. It is known that women who began to menstruate when particularly young or who reached menopause when particularly old develop breast cancer more frequently than other women. On the other hand, among women who have first pregnancies when young, the rate of breast cancer is lower than among women who never bear children or who do so after the age of 30. These patterns in relation to menarche, sexual activity, pregnancy, and menopause implicate differences in levels of sex hormones. Elevated levels of estrogens and other female hormones are associated with higher frequencies of breast cancer.[13] Increased body weight and increased consumption of fat and animal protein are also associated with higher rates of this cancer. Radiation also can cause breast cancer (see Chapter 8); a group of women given X-ray therapy for tuberculosis experienced a 10-fold increase in breast cancer.[14] Chemical carcinogens may also cause some breast cancers (Chapter 7).

To these physiological and environmental factors can be added a hereditary factor. For American women as a group, the overall risk of developing breast cancer is about 1 in 12. But among women who have a blood relative (mother, sister, aunt, or grandmother) with breast cancer, the rate nearly triples, to about 1 in 5. As with other cancers in which heredity plays a role, women with a family history of breast cancer tend to develop this cancer at an earlier age and are more likely to be stricken in both breasts than are women without such a family history. For example, in one family the maternal grandmother developed breast cancer at age 48, the mother had breast cancer at 42, and two daughters developed the cancer at ages 22 and 29. Prophylactic (preventative) mastectomy of both breasts was recommended to a third daughter (age 19) because it seemed extremely likely that she, too, would be stricken.[15]

Somewhat less than 1 percent of all breast cancer occurs in males, and here too hereditary influences are apparent. Three men in one family developed breast cancer. In another family with three cases of male breast cancer, breast cancer was also unusually frequent among female relatives.[15]

The question of how genetic factors may cause breast cancer remains open; again some clues suggest possible answers. It seems clear that many genes affect the quantities of estrogens and other sex-related hormones produced in a person's body. Other genes may affect the sensitivity of each tissue to these hormones. A number of genes are thus implicated in controlling the reproduction and differentiation of breast cells. Mutation of one or another of these genes may induce cells of the breast to leave G1 arrest inappropriately—a cancer-causing mutation (Figure 5 in Chapter 2).

Familial breast cancer may thus involve the inheritance of defects in more than one kind of gene. Whatever the case, what is inherited is a susceptibility to the cancer, a susceptibility that presumably will not be realized unless the dividing cell is exposed to an environmental carcinogen. Note, too, that only a single breast cell needs to suffer a mutation. All of the remaining millions may remain normal, in spite of the fact that they are exposed to the same mix of hormones and to the same environmental carcinogens and are genetically identical to the cell that is converted.

These ideas are consistent with the results of the breeding experiments with mice mentioned at the start of this chapter. It is possible to breed strains of mice that are virtually resistant to virally caused breast cancer and to breed other strains that are very susceptible to the same virus. But mice of the latter strains do not develop breast cancer unless they are exposed to the virus: they inherit a susceptibility to cancer, not the cancer itself.

It is not known whether cancer-causing viruses are involved in human breast cancer, although some evidence points in that direction (Chapter 9). As research unravels the details of human familial breast cancer, it seems plausible to expect to discover that it is the result of an inherited increase in susceptibility to chemical carcinogens, radiation, or a cancer-causing virus.

HEREDITARY FACTORS IN SKIN CANCER

Skin cancer is caused by certain chemical carcinogens and by radiation, for example, X rays and ultraviolet light. In some animals, skin cancer can also be caused by viruses (Chapter 9). Physicians diagnose about 400,000 new cases of skin cancer each year in the United States, and it is becoming more frequent. From 1934 to 1972, the rate of skin cancer in Europe increased by 60 percent. Because most skin cancers do not metastasize readily and because they are usually detected when still small, complete and permanent cures are almost always achieved through either surgery or radiation treatments.

The exceptions to routinely curable skin cancers are melanomas, which are skin cancers that arise from pigmented cells in the skin. Some kinds of melanoma metastasize to other organs in the body even when the primary cancer is still small enough to escape notice.[16] About 35 percent of melanoma patients die of the cancer within 5 years after diagnosis. Fortunately, less than 5 percent of skin cancers are melanomas.[17]

The frequency of skin cancer is closely correlated with exposure to sunlight. Skin cancer, including malignant melanoma, is most frequent in tropical regions and becomes progressively less frequent with distance from the equator. Skin cancer also occurs more frequently in people occupationally exposed to the sun, for example, sailors and farmers, and usually arises in the most exposed parts of the body, namely, the face, back of the neck, hands, and arms. It is now known that light in the ultraviolet (UV) region of the spectrum is most efficient in causing skin cancers.

To understand the nature of skin cancer, it is necessary to understand the structure of the skin (Figure 2). Skin consists of an outer layer, the EPIDERMIS, and an underlying layer, the DERMIS. The epidermis is about 50 cells thick. Only the cells in the deepest (basal) layer reproduce, and these are called STEM CELLS. When one of these stem cells divides, it produces on the average one new stem cell and one cell that moves into the layer immediately above and begins to differentiate. Differentiating skin cells synthesize large amounts of a protein called KERATIN, which makes skin relatively tough and water-

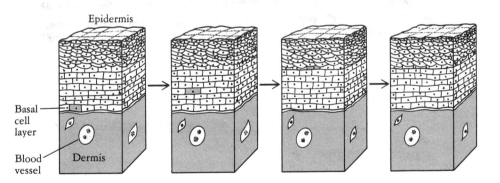

FIGURE 2 Skin cells formed deep in the epidermis differentiate as they are pushed toward the body's surface by younger cells forming beneath them.

proof; hair and nails are almost entirely keratin. As the differentiating epidermal cells are pushed closer to the skin's surface, they become progressively flatter and less vigorous. When fully differentiated, these cells stop dividing and later die as they are cut off from all sources of nutrients. Therefore, cells in the outermost layers of the epidermis are dead and form a tough, protective barrier.

The number of new skin cells added by the dividing stem cells in the basal layer is usually balanced by the sloughing off of dead cells at the skin's surface. On the scalp, dead cells may be sloughed in large clumps (called dandruff). Thus cells in the upper layers of skin are constantly renewed, a process essential for maintaining a healthy skin and for repairing burns, abrasions, and other wounds.

Below the basal layer of the epidermis is the deeper layer of the skin, called the dermis. Certain cells in the dermis known as MELANOCYTES synthesize the pigment MELANIN. Through extensions of the cytoplasm, the melanocytes transfer melanin granules to cells of the basal layer of the epidermis, giving the epidermis its pigmented characteristics. Both the number of melanocytes in a person's skin and the amount of pigment they produce are genetically determined—thus the range of skin coloration from black (many melanocytes) to brown (intermediate number of melanocytes) to pale (few melanocytes).

Most skin cancers begin in the stem cells of the basal layer of the epidermis. For ultraviolet light to cause skin cancer, it must penetrate the layers of dead and differentiating cells and reach the basal layer.[18] The effectiveness with which the basal layer is shielded from the damaging effects of ultraviolet light depends on several inherited characteristics: how thick the epidermis is, how many melanocytes are in the basal layer, and how much melanin they contain. Melanin is important because it absorbs and reflects ultraviolet light and thus shields the stem cells in the basal layer. The more pigment in a person's skin, the less susceptible the person will be to skin cancer. Therefore, skin cancer is much less frequent among deeply pigmented people and increases gradually as skin color becomes progressively paler. Among Caucasians, brunettes have the most melanin, blondes have less, and redheads have the least; susceptibility to skin cancer follows the same pattern. Of course, skin color is modified by exposure to UV light because UV light induces melanocytes to synthesize more melanin (tanning), which increases protection against damage from sunlight. Some people tan more quickly than others, and this too is an inherited characteristic. Inherited susceptibility to skin cancer is thus at least partly a matter of how much melanin a person's skin cells are genetically programmed to synthesize.

The importance of the skin's thickness can be seen in the hand. The skin on the face and on the backs of the neck, hands, and arms is relatively thin and more susceptible to skin cancer than, say, the palm, which is covered by a much thicker layer of dead cells. Indeed, the skin on the palm is so thick that ultraviolet light cannot penetrate sufficiently to induce the synthesis of pigment, and the palm does not ordinarily become tan. As might be expected from this, skin cancer of the palm is very rare.

Among different groups of humans, people who inherit more pigment in their skin also tend to inherit thicker epidermal layers. Thus blacks tend to be doubly protected against the carcinogenic effects of sunlight, and whites (particularly the most fair) inherit a kind of double susceptibility or jeopardy.

Again, note that these inherited differences determine differences in *susceptibility* to skin cancers. A person who inherits pale, thin skin will develop skin cancer only if exposed to a sufficient dose of an environmental carcinogen, say, the sun's rays or a tanning lamp.

Inherited Susceptibility May Result from Defective DNA Repair

A number of genetic disorders in humans clearly result in an increased susceptibility to cancer. These genetic disorders are identified by one or another abnormality in development of a tissue or organ before the appearance of cancer. Almost always the abnormalities occur in childhood, although in some cases the associated health problems come in young adulthood. Fortunately these hereditary conditions are quite rare. Some are better understood than others.

In the exceedingly rare genetic disorder known as XERODERMA PIGMENTOSUM, the skin of an affected individual is hypersensitive to sunlight. The skin becomes freckled and blisters easily. More seriously, multiple, separate, malignant skin tumors develop. Most affected individuals die before they reach 20 years of age.

Individuals afflicted with xeroderma pigmentosum received a defective copy of a particular gene from *each* parent. This gene normally codes for a protein that repairs the kind of damage to DNA caused by ultraviolet light. Lacking a normal copy of this gene, the skin cells of a person with xeroderma pigmentosum are unable to repair UV-damaged DNA. Therefore, mutations accumulate at an abnormally high rate in the skin cells. Inevitably, mutations occur in one or more genes whose functions are essential for normal control of G1 arrest. Such a mutated cell may initiate a skin cancer.

To avoid almost certain skin cancer, persons with this genetic disorder must scrupulously avoid all ultraviolet light, which means absolute protection from direct sunlight. In one case of identical twins with xeroderma pigmentosum, a cancer-control program consisting of complete avoidance of UV light (protective clothing, dark glasses, photoprotective lotion, etc.) has succeeded to the extent that both twins have reached their late teens without any evidence of cancer.[15] One, however, recently began to smoke cigarettes, a behavior that might prove fatal (see Chapter 7).

Another rare inherited disorder, Fanconi's anemia, is characterized by underproduction of red blood cells (hence the anemia) and by an increase in the number of broken chromosomes, particularly in white blood cells. The broken chromosomes suggest a defect in the normal capacity to repair breaks in DNA. The increase in broken chromosomes is in some way related to the fact that persons with Fanconi's anemia often develop leukemia. Victims usually die at an early age.[19]

There is a variety of other rare genetic disorders such as Bloom's syndrome, ataxia telangiectasia, multiple neurofibromatosis, and nevoid basal cell carcinoma syndrome.   Together, all such cancers caused by genetic disorders constitute a small fraction (less than 1 percent) of all cancers. Their rarity is of little solace to the victims and their families. In the context of the total problem of cancer, however, studying these rare diseases may provide valuable, basic information about the genetic basis of cancer in general, information that may lead to an understanding of the causes of other, far more prevalent forms of cancer.

Such insights have already come from studies of the more common familial cancers. It is established, for example, that susceptibility to cancer, not the disease itself, is inherited. Moreover, familial susceptibility may take any of several forms. In at least one case (hereditary retinoblastoma), the susceptibility seems to involve the inheritance of a defective regulatory gene. In others, susceptibility involves inheritance of anatomical or physiological features, as in skin cancer and breast cancer. In xeroderma pigmentosum, the susceptibility reflects the malfunction of a defective repair enzyme; this malfunction permits the accumulation of mutations—some, presumably, among regulatory genes.

In many, perhaps most, cancers, the immediate causal event may be a mutation that impairs normal controls over the effectiveness of G1 arrest. Cells inappropriately released from normal controls over reproduction are often cancerous. These and other examples emphasize the diversity of what might otherwise be regarded as a single disease and also shape the discussions of the next four chapters dealing with the agents that induce cancers.

6

Environment and Cancer

ALTHOUGH cancer has afflicted humans since earliest times, it was a rare disease until the twentieth century (Chapter 1). Lung cancer, which now causes 1 of every 20 deaths in the United States, was so rare that many nineteenth century physicians never encountered a single case during an entire professional career. And until relatively recently, cancer was viewed fatalistically, as an inescapable malady. In contrast, it is now known that most, perhaps almost all, cancers are caused by factors in our environment. In this context, our environment includes everything with which we may in one way or another come into routine contact: air, water, food, and clothing; sunlight, X rays, and other radiations; viruses; drugs, medicines, pesticides, herbicides, dyes, preservatives, cigarette smoke, asbestos, and a myriad of other chemicals in common use. This vast range of environmental factors can be conveniently grouped into three general categories, namely, chemicals, radiations, and viruses. Each of the next three chapters is devoted to the major, specific carcinogens in one of these categories and to what is known about how specific carcinogens cause cancer. Most carcinogens are introduced into the environment by human activities and are therefore controllable or removable, at least in principle. Consequently, removing or at least avoiding environmental carcinogens offers the opportunity to prevent most cancers.

Environmental Carcinogens Were Known Two Centuries Ago

Links between the environment and the occurrence of particular kinds of cancer were first recognized more than 200 years ago. In 1761, Dr. John Hill, a London physician, published his conclusion that snuff (powdered tobacco) caused nasal cancer. He included the admonition,

With respect to cancers of the nose, they are as dreadful and as fatal as any others. . . . It is evident therefore that no man should venture upon Snuff, who is not sure that he is not so far liable to a cancer: and no man can be sure of that.[1]

Inhaling snuff through the nose is now uncommon but taking snuff orally, between cheek and gum, is becoming increasingly popular. Women in the rural southern United States have long used tobacco snuff in this way and have long been prone to an oral cancer known locally as "snuff dipper's cancer."[2] The growing use of "smokeless tobacco" will in time inevitably lead to an increase in oral cancers.

In 1775, the British physician Percivall Pott published his observations on the high incidence of scrotal cancer among men who had been chimney sweeps as youngsters.[3] Soot from incompletely burned coal tended to lodge in the folds of the scrotal skin of young sweeps. Carcinogens in the soot dissolved in the natural oils of scrotal skin, causing what came to be called "soot-wart" or "chimney-sweeper's cancer." Subsequently, when Danish chimney sweeps were required to wear protective clothing and to wash regularly, the frequency of this cancer decreased among them. The case of scrotal cancer in chimney sweeps not only provides an early example of environmental carcinogenesis, but also was the first successful program of cancer prevention.

These 200-year-old lessons have been largely ignored. Coke-oven workers in the United States steel industry suffer from a rate of fatal lung cancer that is ten times higher than in steel workers not involved with coke ovens.[4] Coke ovens generate fumes that contain carcinogenic substances similar to those that caused chimney sweep's cancer. It has been known for more than a century that similar carcinogens cause cancers among coal-tar and shale-oil workers. Yet thousands of coke-oven workers today are exposed to these same kinds of carcinogens in their work environments.

In 1820, a high incidence of scrotal cancer was described among copper smelters who were occupationally exposed to arsenic compounds. More recently, people exposed to arsenic have been found to suffer higher rates of cancers of the skin, lung, lymphatic system, and liver. Yet large numbers of Americans and Europeans continue to be exposed in their jobs to similar kinds of arsenic compounds. In 1895, aromatic amines were found to cause bladder cancers in dye workers; yet many American workers are still being exposed to certain amines such as benzidine. Fifty percent of the former employees of one United States benzidine plant were reported to have developed bladder cancer. In 1894, the unusual frequency of skin cancers among sailors was correctly attributed to their long exposure to sunlight; yet today millions sunbathe excessively and thousands pay to rent "tanning parlors." Radioactive substances such as uranium isotopes have been known for over 50 years to cause lung cancer and possibly other kinds of cancers, yet uranium miners still inhale radioactive dusts today.

These are a few examples of the early recognition of associations between certain environmental agents and certain kinds of cancer. These were among the first demonstrations of environmental carcinogenesis in general and of occupational carcinogenesis in particular. One might wonder why such early discoveries did not lead to a broader understanding that most, or even all, kinds of cancers might be caused by environmental agents. Part of the explanation is that the many different kinds of cancers that occur in different tissues were originally viewed as quite different diseases, with little if any relation to one another. Only relatively recently was the common feature of all cancers recognized to be a defect(s) in normal regulation of cell differentiation and cell division. This major theoretical advance enabled researchers to see cancers as a set of related diseases. In turn, this permitted the pooling of research on the causes and treatments of cancers, accelerating the growth of understanding and of subsequent research.

Carcinogens Can Be Recognized and Identified

The discovery of most human carcinogens involved careful observations and simple cause-and-effect logic. When an unusual proportion of a particular group of people (chimney sweeps, coke workers, sailors, or uranium miners) develop some particular form of cancer, suspicions are raised and efforts are made to identify a causal factor common to that group. Thus, coal soot was identified as the common factor among chimney sweeps, coke fumes among coke workers, sunlight among sailors, and radioactive dusts among uranium miners. This kind of logic is the basis of the epidemiological method of searching for carcinogens: one tries to correlate an unusual pattern of cancers with some environmental, life-style, or genetic pattern.

An important example of the epidemiological study of cancer involved the drastic increase, which was first noticed a few decades ago, in the incidence of lung cancer among United States males (Figure 7C in Chapter 1). Analyses of this epidemic revealed that most lung cancer victims had one environmental component in common: cigarette smoke. Not all cigarette smokers were developing lung cancers and not all victims of lung cancer were smokers. But cigarette smokers as a group were suffering far more lung cancers than nonsmokers as a group.[5] Correlations of that sort suggested that smoking cigarettes could cause lung cancer; correlational evidence of that sort is merely circumstantial. Proof that cigarette smoke does, in fact, contain materials that cause lung cancer came from other sources. Epidemiologists established that heavy smokers more often developed lung cancer than did light smokers, that long-term smokers more often developed cancer than did short-term smokers. Laboratory scientists demonstrated that cigarette smoke does cause cancer in laboratory animals under controlled conditions.[5] Pure carcinogens were eventually isolated from cigarette smoke (Chapter 7). Proofs of these kinds are now overwhelming. The search for such proofs was, in the first instance, prompted by early epidemiological correlations.

Almost all of the 35 or so proved human carcinogens were first implicated by epidemiological studies.[6] Such studies continue to alert us to the possibility of as-yet-unrecognized environmental carcinogens. Recent epidemiological studies confirm that various cancers occur at vastly different rates in different regions of the world and among people with different styles of living. Esophageal cancer, for example, occurs at an extraordinarily high rate in northeast Iran, eventually striking about one in five persons who live to the age of 75.[7] Stomach cancer is unusually frequent in Japan, rectal cancer is high in Denmark, and breast cancer is higher in the United States than in most other regions of the world. Explanations for these differences are not yet developed.[2] Hereditary differences can generally be ruled out (see Chapter 5), indicating that environmental agents cause at least some of these epidemiological patterns.

However useful it has been in the past, the epidemiological approach to detecting environmental carcinogens is limited. Epidemiological data are, at least initially, little more than circumstantial evidence, but do provide reasons for initiating a search for possible carcinogens. Vast differences in heredity, in personal histories, and in life-styles, even within a small community, confound searches for epidemiological patterns and correlations. The fact that most human cancers result from many insults sustained over long periods makes the search even more difficult, especially in the absence of reliable lifetime medical and occupational histories. Epidemiological methods are also relatively insensitive. The rate of a particular cancer in a given subpopulation must be considerably higher than that in the general population in order for the difference to be detectable. Finally, epidemiological insights, often gained by analyzing death certificates and other public health records, are tragically retrospective, often by decades.

These and other limitations argue that although we must continue to gather epidemiological data and to act on leads they offer, epidemiology alone is inadequate, and that additional sources of data about potential carcinogens are also needed.

TESTING CARCINOGENS WITH ANIMALS

Epidemiological evidence that some environmental factor is a human carcinogen is only presumptive—a first step. A suspected carcinogen must be evaluated in other ways, for example, by exposing animals to it in experiments designed to determine whether indeed it does cause cancer, under what circumstances, and at what doses. Some substances cause cancer when taken into an animal in a single, minute dose; other carcinogens cause cancer only after prolonged exposures to relatively massive doses.

Hundreds of carcinogens have been identified by exposing test animals to suspected substances.[8] Some were suggested by epidemiological studies, others were not. What leads a researcher to suspect that one or another substance might be a carcinogen is discussed in the next chapter. The point is that it is not necessary to carry out unintended, long-term "experiments" on ourselves and our environment to identify carcinogens. Instead, it is possible to use laboratory animals to identify carcinogens already in the environment as well as to recognize in advance carcinogens that might otherwise be unwittingly introduced into the environment, only to be "discovered" decades later on an epidemiologically detectable scale.

The advantages of using laboratory animals to screen potential carcinogens are similar to those realized by using them in genetic studies (Chapter 5). Laboratory animals have short life spans, can be maintained under rigidly controlled conditions, and can be subjected to any convenient program of exposure to potential carcinogens. Most importantly, tests with animals can be done prospectively, before large quantities of newly synthesized substances are disseminated into our environment.

The logic behind animal tests is simple (Figure 1). A population of identical animals is divided into a number of groups. Each group is exposed to some controlled dose of the suspected

(A)   Groups of identical test animals

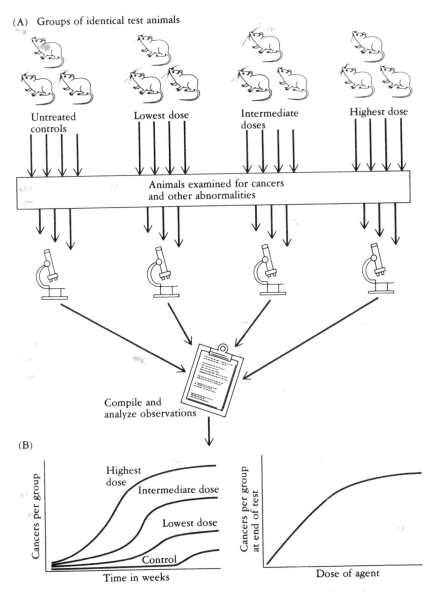

FIGURE 1   Using laboratory animals to test suspected carcinogens. (A) Groups of identical animals are exposed to various doses of the agent being tested. As animals die, they are examined for cancers. Surviving animals are killed and similarly examined at the end of the test. (B) Graphs summarizing data from a hypothetical test of a carcinogen.

carcinogen, at some standard rate, for some predetermined period. In practice, doses usually range from zero (controls) to the maximum nonlethal quantity tolerated by the animals. At some later time the animals are killed and their cells and tissues examined for cancers, damaged chromosomes, and other abnormalities. A judgment is then made as to whether or not the suspected carcinogen induced a significant number of abnormalities.

Evaluating potential carcinogens through animal tests thus is direct but unfortunately not problem-free; few approaches are. A basic unresolved issue concerns the validity of extrapolating to the human situation findings that are made with laboratory animals. For example, are substances that prove to be carcinogenic in laboratory animals *necessarily* carcinogenic to humans? Almost all of the substances that are known to cause cancer in humans do also cause cancer in animals.[6] Therefore it seems reasonable to expect that carcinogens discovered in animals may also be carcinogenic in humans. There are, however, occasional exceptions. For example, it is established beyond doubt that arsenic causes skin and lung cancer and probably lymphatic and liver cancer in humans,[9] but it has not yet been possible to demonstrate that arsenic causes cancer in certain other animals. Similarly, the substance 2-acetylaminofluorene (AAF) is a powerful carcinogen in rats but does not cause cancer in guinea pigs. The reason for this difference in susceptibility has been thoroughly studied and is now well understood: AAF is a precarcinogen (see below); rat tissues contain enzymes that convert AAF to a carcinogen; guinea pig tissues do not. AAF would almost certainly be a carcinogen for humans (as it is for most animals) because human tissues contain the enzymes for its conversion. The first evidence that the substance is carcinogenic in animals was reported in 1941.[10] The U.S. Occupational Safety and Health Administration finally regulated industrial exposure of humans to this compound in 1973, at a time when the chemical industry was preparing to produce massive amounts of the substance for use as an insecticide.[11]

Problems raised by such differences among species can in

part be avoided by testing a suspected carcinogen in two or more species. Other issues concerning the extrapolation of animal tests to humans are less easily resolved. To make animal tests maximally powerful, very high doses of the suspected factor are employed, doses proportionally much higher than a person might reasonably encounter. Similarly, many tests are done with strains of animals specifically bred to be susceptible to certain kinds of cancers. Such practices may therefore overestimate the hazards to humans. On the other hand, it is well known that some chemicals, although not themselves carcinogens, enhance the potency of many chemicals that are carcinogens (see Chapter 7). These are called COCARCINOGENS. The identification of these compounds supports the belief that much human cancer results from the combined effects of several environmental insults. Therefore animal tests may underestimate the hazards to humans. These and other issues concerning the theory and interpretation of animal tests for carcinogens are discussed further in Chapter 11. The conclusion here (and there) is that potential environmental carcinogens can be identified *prospectively* through tests with laboratory animals, although not always unequivocally. Agents so identified must be regarded, at least potentially, as contributors to environmentally induced human cancer.

SHORT-TERM TESTS FOR CARCINOGENS

Although prospective, animal tests are relatively insensitive and neither inexpensive nor rapid. Testing a single chemical in a single species may cost in excess of $400,000 and may occupy several scientists and technicians for 2 years or longer. Thousands of chemicals have been added to the environment over the last half-century. As discussed later, the number and amount of these has increased enormously since 1950: motor vehicle exhaust and other wastes of fossil fuels; industrial wastes in water and air; preservatives and other food additives; herbicides, pesticides, and other agricultural chemicals. Some of these substances have been shown to be carcinogenic through testing in animals, usually mice. Literally thousands of other chemicals already disseminated in the environment and tens of thousands of new chemicals proposed for future use remain to be tested. Given that testing the carcinogenicity of a single chemical in animals requires at least several hundreds of thousands of dollars and 2 or more years, the task of testing so many chemicals seems impractical.

During the past decade, a number of short-term tests have been developed that overcome the shortcomings of animal tests. These short-term tests use bacteria or other unicellular organisms or mammalian cells growing in artificial media as test organisms. Such tests are based on the observation that many agents capable of causing mutations are also capable of causing cancer.[12] Evidence that supports this connection accumulated slowly during decades of basic research in genetics and cell biology. Indeed, the central messages of Chapters 3 and 4 are (1) that cancer results from mutations induced in genes that normally regulate the reproduction and differentiation of cells and (2) that mutations in all organisms involve fundamentally similar chemical processes. *So many mutagens do, in fact, cause cancer that the mutagenicity of an agent is presumptive evidence that the agent may also cause cancer.* It is quite conceivable that *all* mutagens are carcinogens and that the present inability to demonstrate this for some mutagens is due to the insensitivity of animal tests that must be used to confirm carcinogenicity.

The original and still most widely used short-term test is called the AMES TEST after its originator, a biochemist at the University of California at Berkeley. The Ames test measures the capacity of a chemical to cause mutations in special strains of the bacterium *Salmonella typhimurium. S. typhimurium* is well understood at the biochemical and genetic levels and is well suited for tests of mutagenicity. Ames and his colleagues developed several strains of *S. typhimurium* that carry mutations that render the cells incapable of synthesizing the amino acid histidine. Such cells, called histidine-minus mutants, grow and multiply perfectly well in medium containing histidine but cannot do so in medium from which histidine is missing. Histidine-minus mutants may regain the ability to synthesize histidine as the result of normally rare, secondary mutations, called BACK MUTATIONS. Cells that sustain such back mutations will, of course, be able to grow and multiply in media from which histidine is missing; this is the basis of the Ames test (Figure 2).[13]

Hundreds of millions of histidine-minus cells are grown in a medium containing histidine, then transferred to culture dishes of medium lacking only histidine. A small quantity of the chemical being tested is also added to the culture dishes. If the chemical is a mutagen for *S. typhimurium*, it will induce many kinds of mutations in many of the cells. At least some of these will be back mutations that restore the capacity to synthesize histidine. Each cell that sustains such a mutation will grow and multiply, giving rise in a day or so to a visible colony of cells. The number of such colonies will reflect the mutagenicity of the chemical, the amount used, and other variables that can be readily controlled and standardized.

Such bacterial tests are extraordinarily sensitive, take only a few days to complete, and cost only a few hundred dollars per chemical. Unfortunately, they are not foolproof. Many chemicals are not carcinogenic as they occur in the environment but become carcinogenic only after undergoing biochemical changes within a cell.[14] The chemical benzo[a]pyrene provides a case in point. This substance occurs in motor vehicle exhaust, smoke from fossil fuels, tobacco smoke, charcoal-broiled foods, and in many industrial processes; it is currently one of the most important hazards found in the human environment.[15] Benzo[a]pyrene does not induce mutations in bacterial tests and it is not in itself directly carcinogenic. However, benzo[a]pyrene is converted through normal metabolic reactions in mammalian cells into a variety of other compounds, some of which are both strongly mutagenic and carcinogenic.[16] Therefore benzo[a]pyrene appropriately is considered to be an environmental carcinogen even though it is not mutagenic in bacterial tests like the Ames test.

So it is with many other chemicals: they are not mutagenic or carcinogenic as they occur in the environment but become so only after "metabolic activation" in mammalian cells. In general, metabolic activation of precarcinogens into carcinogens is the result of the action of certain enzymes that normally function to destroy poisons (for example, ethyl alcohol) that enter the cell. Unfortunately these enzymes also bring about chemical changes that convert harmless precarcinogens into

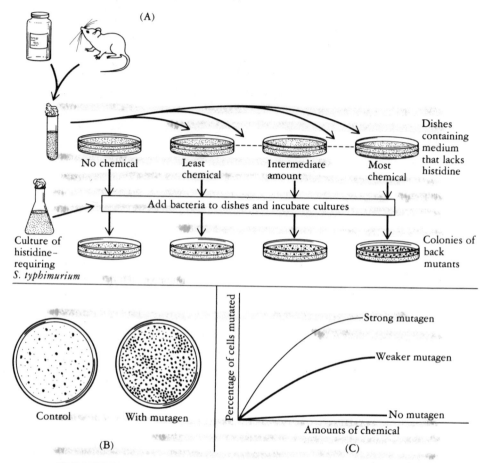

FIGURE 2 Principle of the Ames test for mutagens. (A) The chemical being tested is incubated with homogenized liver and graded amounts of the mixture are dispensed into dishes containing a culture medium that lacks histidine. Bacteria that cannot grow without histidine are added to the dishes and incubated. Cells that sustain certain kinds of back mutations regain the capacity to synthesize histidine, grow, and form visible colonies after 1–2 days. The frequency of such colonies is a measure of the chemical's potency as a mutagen. (B) Culture dishes from an Ames test. The plate on the left is a control (no chemical), that on the right contains a mutagen as shown by the colonies of back mutants. (C) A graph that compares results from hypothetical Ames tests on three chemicals.

potent carcinogens. Ordinarily beneficial enzymes thus become liabilities when we encounter precarcinogens, for example, benzo[a]pyrene. Bacteria do not form these detoxification enzymes. As a result, precarcinogens are generally not mutagenic in bacterial tests because they are not converted to the active forms. For this reason, potential carcinogens being screened in bacterial test systems are first mixed with a suspension of ground-up mammalian cells (usually liver) that contain a mixture of detoxification enzymes.

Another problem is that bacterial tests have failed to demonstrate the mutagenicity of some proved carcinogens, for example, the human carcinogens arsenic and various metal salts.[17] Presumably this kind of failure might happen because of expectable differences between bacteria and mammals in sensitivity to these chemicals or because the tissue extracts used did not contain an appropriate enzyme to convert the chemical into its mutagenic form. In any case, the exceptions seem too few to contradict the principle that most mutagens are also carcinogens.[18] Additional improvements and refinements that remove such exceptions are likely to emerge from additional experiences with bacterial screening tests of the Ames type.

Even now, however, such short-term tests are an important way to recognize many chemical mutagens—affordably and in a timely way. These recognized mutagens can then be subjected to slower, more costly prospective tests in animals to determine if they are, in fact, carcinogens as well. For the time being, however, simple prudence dictates avoidance of any substance that causes mutations in bacteria. Some might turn out not to be carcinogenic in humans, only mutagenic, but we should avoid exposing ourselves and our children to mutagens in any case. Mutagens clearly are responsible for a variety of hereditary disorders (diseases) among humans.

Much Environmentally Caused Cancer Can Be Prevented

Together the three sources of information about environmental carcinogens discussed here—epidemiology, tests with laboratory animals, and screening in bacterial systems—all deliver the same message. This message is that although many carcinogenic agents have already been identified, many others remain to be recognized. This leads us back to questions raised in Chapter 1: How much of human cancer is caused by environmental agents? How many of these agents can be eliminated or avoided? And crucially, how much of human cancer might be preventable?

Estimates of how much human cancer is caused by environmental agents range from 70 to 90 percent.[19] Indeed, in the United States alone, using tobacco and its products accounts for over 30 percent of all human cancer and perhaps another 20 percent results from occupational exposures to carcinogens.[20] More precise estimates will eventually come from combinations of epidemiological, biological, biochemical, and genetic studies, but a figure approaching 90 percent now appears plausible. If this estimate proves to be even approximately correct, we can look forward to preventing a very large proportion of all human cancers by eliminating the environmental agents that cause the disease.

How many environmental carcinogens could be eliminated from the environment or otherwise controlled or avoided can be judged only after the nature and sources of the carcinogens are discovered. Almost all of the carcinogens so far discovered could be eliminated or avoided, for example, tobacco and occupational carcinogens. Given that these are responsible for perhaps up to half of all cancers in the United States, eliminating them would presumably halve the incidence of cancer. How much more cancer could be prevented remains to be determined through future research. The problems are to identify the carcinogens, to devise means of eliminating or avoiding them, and then to implement programs that will accomplish that goal.

The next three chapters outline current knowledge of the nature and distribution of the major kinds of human carcinogens—knowledge that will ultimately form the basis for programs to prevent cancer.

7

Chemicals
and Cancer

PERCIVALL Pott deduced in 1775 that coal soot caused scrotal cancer among men who, as boys, had been chimney sweeps.[1] This first recognition of an occupational cancer was followed in the nineteenth century by discoveries of several other associations between occupation and cancer. In particular, by 1900 it had been well established that skin cancer occurs more frequently among workers in the coal tar and pitch industries.[2] Coal tar is an important source of organic solvents (such as benzene, toluene, and xylene) as well as of phenols, creosols, and creosote oils; naphthalenes; and many aniline dyes, which are still widely used. Many of these substances are now proved to be carcinogens.[3]

These early circumstantial observations naturally prompted attempts to confirm the capacity of coal tar and its derivatives to cause cancer. The method used was to apply coal tars to the skins of experimental animals with the expectation of inducing skin cancers. Early efforts of this kind failed, mainly because the exposures were too short. In 1915, two Japanese researchers reported the first induced skin cancers: they had patiently painted the skins of rabbits with coal tars over many months.[4] This success was soon followed by efforts to identify the actual cancer-causing agent(s) in coal tars.

Thus began the study of the induction of cancer with chemicals, a field that has grown enormously and has led to the identification of hundreds of cancer-causing chemicals. To this day, correlations between cancer and occupations, habits, and life-styles continue to give important clues about additional potentially carcinogenic chemicals.

Prolonged Exposure to Chemical Carcinogens Causes Cancer

An extraordinarily important aspect of chemical carcinogenesis is the long delay between the start of more or less continuous contact with the carcinogen and the appearance of the disease. For humans the delay is usually a matter of years and can be as long as 40 years. Cancers caused by tobacco smoke ordinarily develop only after many years of smoking but may occasionally develop after as few as 10 years, or they may never develop at all. These are statistical observations; predictions are impossible for individual smokers.

On the other hand, short exposure to extremely powerful carcinogens can be effective, especially at high doses. The chemical 4-aminobiphenyl, which was manufactured in the United States from 1935 to 1955, is a potent inducer of bladder cancer. More than 18 percent of those occupationally exposed to 4-aminobiphenyl developed bladder cancers. Several persons who subsequently developed bladder cancers were exposed for less than 2 years, and one person was exposed for only 133 days.[5] Among workers exposed to the related compounds benzidine and 2-napthylamine, over 90 percent developed bladder cancer when exposed for 5 years or longer.[6]

The years of delay before a cancer appears are a mixed blessing. Clearly, individuals benefit by escaping cancer as long as possible. On the other hand, the delay greatly complicates the task of eventually identifying a carcinogen. Moreover, the identification then comes too late for many more people who in the meantime have unknowingly been exposed to the carcinogen. Tobacco smoke was identified as a cause of lung and other kinds of cancers only many decades after cigarette smoking had become popular. The discovery was prompted by the epidemiological observation that smokers suffer much higher rates of lung cancer and higher rates of other kinds of cancers.[7] This "test" on unwitting human subjects subsequently led to direct identification of the carcinogens in tobacco smoke (see later). Unfortunately, such "tests" on people continue and at least some involve substances already well documented as potent carcinogens in animals. Other ongoing tests involve substances not yet recognized as carcinogens. In any case, it can be said that this long latency period means that cancers that arise today largely result from carcinogens that have been in our environment for the last 20 to 40 years. And the cancer-causing agents added to our environment today will reveal their effects as cancers that will be seen, for the most part, 20 to 40 years from now.

Initiation and Promotion in Cancer

It is now known that the long delay occurs because the conversion of a normal cell to a cancerous one involves several steps. These steps occur in two stages called initiation and promotion. INITIATION occurs when cells are exposed to a limited dose, even a single dose, of a carcinogenic substance. An initiated cell usually does not develop into a cancer cell without some further alteration. Cells that have undergone initiation are not generally recognizable as such, although in a few kinds of tissues initiated cells may have a slightly abnormal appearance. Initiation is irreversible, and initiated cells disappear only by dying. Also, when an initiated cell divides, both of its daughters inherit the initiated state. Much evidence indicates that initiation is the result of mutation, an idea consistent with the irreversible nature of the process and the inheritance of the state. An initiated cell may be converted into a cancer cell by subsequent exposure to an initiator in a second process called promotion. PROMOTION may be achieved by exposure to the same initiator that caused the initiation *or* to another initiator. Those agents that can both initiate *and* promote cancer are called COMPLETE CARCINOGENS.

The point is that cancer-causing agents often work together, one causing initiation and another causing promotion. For example, uranium miners who smoke are exposed to multiple initiators and promoters: the radioactivity of uranium and various chemicals in cigarette smoke. Because their effects are additive, a uranium miner who also smokes has a 4-fold greater risk of lung cancer than a smoking nonminer and almost a 100-fold greater risk than a nonsmoking nonminer.[8]

Some substances cannot cause initiation but can promote an initiated cell into a cancer. Asbestos appears to be such a promoter because it alone probably does not cause cancer. Rather, exposure to asbestos increases the rate of lung cancer among smokers 8-fold.[9] Cigarette smoke, which contains several initiators (as well as promoters), initiates cells that can be promoted to cancer cells by subsequent exposure to asbestos. Currently there are in the United States over one million persons who have had, or are now subject to, prolonged occupational exposure to asbestos. Asbestos is also used in the manufacture of many common and widely used consumer goods, including a spray-on ceiling insulation common in public buildings such as schools. Asbestos has become such a common airborne pollutant in the United States that it occurs in the lungs of more than 80 percent of Americans who are not occupationally exposed to it.[10] Asbestos may also be an important promoter of cancer in cells initiated by carcinogens other than those of cigarette smoke, for example, the carcinogens in polluted urban air. If so, an epidemic of asbestos-promoted cancers some decades hence may yet be witnessed.

In short, formation of a cancer cell begins with an initiating event that is probably a mutation that may occur after only brief exposure to an initiator. Conversion of an initiated cell to a cancer cell (promotion) usually requires subsequent prolonged, repeated exposure to a promoting agent. This stage may account for most of the lag in induction of cancer. The action of promoters remains unclear, but some evidence suggests that they too mutate genes or damage chromosomes.

The delay between the exposure to initiators and promoters and the appearance of cancer also depends on a number of additional factors, particularly intensity of the exposures. A person who smokes 40 cigarettes per day is not only more likely to get lung cancer than someone who smokes 20 cigarettes per day but is also likely to develop lung cancer sooner. An example with animals illustrates the point more precisely. *All* of a group of mice exposed to small doses of the coal tar derivative dibenzanthracene developed cancer with an average delay of just over 5 months. Another group exposed to doses 16 times larger developed cancer with an average delay of just over 3.5 months—1.5 months sooner.

Cancers Are Probably Caused by Mutagens

Many allusions were made earlier to a relationship between carcinogenesis and mutation, and this section presents briefly some evidence of the relationship. Because the cancer property is inherited through cell division by all of the progeny of a cancer cell, it has long been suspected that a cancer cell carries defective genes that account for its cancerous behavior. The identification of specific cancer-causing chemicals ultimately led to a direct test of this idea.

A great deal has been learned about mutation-causing chemicals, MUTAGENS, largely through studies on microorganisms and particularly on bacteria, and the general properties of mutagens have been defined. For example, mutagens have chemical properties that allow them to interact with DNA in such a way that at the point of interaction on the long DNA molecule a chemical change constituting a mutation may occur (Figure 1). Most carcinogens have chemical properties that lead one to suspect that they are also mutagenic. The suspicion is borne out by direct tests of their mutagenicity on bacteria. Bacteria are used because the mutagenic potency of a chemical can be accurately, simply, and inexpensively measured in tests based on the Ames test (Chapter 6). Such tests can also be done using human or other mammalian cells growing in culture, but this latter procedure is more difficult, takes more time, and is more expensive. However, substances that are mutagenic for bacteria also are usually mutagenic for human cells, although occasional exceptions occur.

Comparisons of tests with bacteria and with animals support

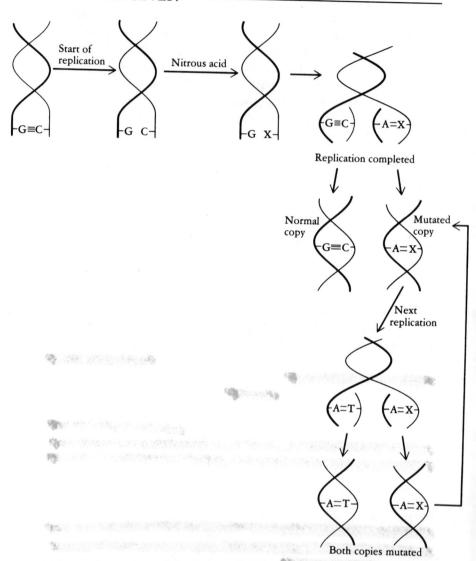

FIGURE 1 An example of chemically caused point mutations. Nitrous acid converts the base C into a base X, which pairs with the base A. When they replicate, GX pairs produce mutated DNAs containing AX pairs in place of GC pairs. When AX pairs replicate, they form two types of mutated DNAs: DNAs in which an original GC pair is now replaced by an AT pair; and DNAs in which an original GC pair is replaced by an AX pair.

three generalizations. (1) About 90 percent of the hundreds of substances known to be carcinogenic initiators in animals cause mutations in bacteria. (2) Substances that do not cause mutations in bacteria generally fail to act as initiators when tested in animals, although again a few exceptions have been found. (3) Chemicals that are found to be mutagenic in bacteria have always proved to be complete carcinogens when thoroughly tested in animals.[11] Thus, it may be concluded that most carcinogens (initiators) are mutagens and that all mutagens are probably carcinogens.

Tobacco Causes Cancer

Tobacco was used by native Americans long before the arrival of Europeans. The drug was introduced into Europe about 1558, and by 1620 tobacco had become a major crop in Virginia. Its production and use have increased steadily to this day. In 1976, the worldwide tobacco crop amounted to 5.5 million tons, which went into 3.85 trillion cigarettes as well as into cigars, pipe tobacco, snuff, and other products.[12,13]

In 1761, the London physician John Hill reported an association between the use of tobacco snuff and nasal cancer.[14] In 1795, a report of an increased incidence of lip cancer in pipe smokers was published.[15] The systematic study of the relationship between the use of tobacco and disease did not begin in earnest, however, until the 1930s, three centuries after its use had become common.

It is now known that the use of tobacco (largely cigarette smoking) is a major contributor to (1) cardiovascular diseases, (2) noncancerous respiratory diseases such as chronic bronchitis, emphysema, and chronic obstructive lung disease, (3) peptic ulcer disease, and (4) cancer, including cancers of the lung, larynx, mouth, esophagus, bladder, kidneys, and pancreas. Among male smokers, the overall death rate is about double that of nonsmokers for all ages between 35 and 74. Over the age of 74, smokers have only about a 25 percent greater death rate. Cigarette smokers experience about 40 percent more lost work days due to illness than nonsmokers. This is equivalent to a total excess loss of over 80 million work days per year in the United States. The economic loss in the form of premature death, health costs, and work loss is equivalent to tens of billions of dollars every year in the United States alone, to say nothing of the toll in avoidable health problems and human misery.

The effect of cigarette smoking on life expectancy for United States males is shown in Figure 2. The greatest loss of

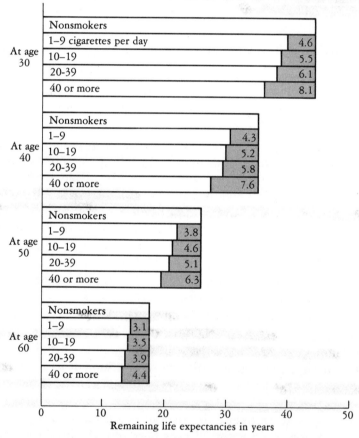

FIGURE 2 Estimated remaining life expectancies for United States males at various ages according to number of cigarettes smoked daily. Shaded bars represent number of years by which life expectancies are reduced by smoking.[16]

years of life is suffered by persons 30 years old or younger who smoke 40 or more cigarettes per day (average of 8.1 years lost), although even those 30-year-olds who smoke fewer than 10 cigarettes a day have their lives shortened by 4.6 years on the average. This decrease in average life expectancy is, of course, a measure of premature deaths among these men.

Currently in the United States, about 38 percent of all males are smokers (down from 53 percent in 1964) and about 29 percent of all females are smokers (down 2 percent since 1964). The most ominous source of new smokers is among teenagers. In the age group of 12–18 years, about 16 percent of boys smoked in 1978 (up 1 percent from 1968) as did 15 percent of girls (up 8 percent from 1968).[7] Many of these teenagers establish lifelong smoking habits that will impair their health and ultimately shorten their lives. It seems likely that the earlier in life a person begins to smoke cigarettes, the greater the expected reduction in life expectancy; however, relevant data are not yet available.

Tobacco smoke is a complex mixture of about 2000 different substances, only some of which have been tested as mutagens. About 50 of these are already proved to be carcinogens (Table 1). The urine of cigarette smokers contains substances that are mutagenic for bacteria and also substances that cause changes in the chromosomes of human cells growing in culture; presumably, these substances in urine are the basis for the higher rate of bladder cancer in cigarette smokers (see below). In addition to carcinogens, cigarette smoke contains other well-known poisons, such as cyanide, cresols, and carbon monoxide; indeed, carbon monoxide is a major component, making up 1 to 5 percent by volume of the smoke. Tobacco smoke also contains significant amounts of several radioactive substances, primarily thorium-228, radium-226, and polonium-210, which may be important in tobacco carcinogenesis (see Chapter 8).[7] Nicotine appears to be the primary incentive for the smoking habit. Nicotine is now considered to be strongly addictive and is likely to be the reason that cigarette smoking is so difficult to give up.

Lung cancer is the leading form of cancer attributable to

TABLE 1. Some of the 2000 chemicals in cigarette smoke. Asterisks (*) mark proved carcinogens.[7]

Acetaldehyde	Fluorene
Acetone	Formaldehyde
Acetylene	Hexane
Acrolein	Hydrazine
Aminostilbene*	Indeno[1,2,3-*cd*]pyrene*
Ammonia	Indole
Arsenic*	Isoprene
Benz[*a*]anthracene*	Methane
Benz[*a*]pyrene*	Methanol
Benzene*	Methylcarbazole
Benzo[*b*]fluoranthene*	5-Methylchrysene*
Benzo[*c*]phenanthrene*	Methylfluoranthene*
Benzo[*j*]fluoranthene	Methylindole
Cadmium*	β-Naphthylamine*
Carbazole	Nickel compounds*
Carbon dioxide	Nicotine
Carbon monoxide	Nitric oxide
Chrysene*	Nitrobenzene
Cresols	Nitroethane
Crotonaldehyde	Nitromethane
Cyanide	N-Nitrosodimethylamine*
DDT	N-Nitrosomethylethylamine*
Dibenz[*a,c*]anthracene*	N-Nitrosodiethylamine*
Dibenzo[*a,e*]fluoranthene*	Nitrosonornicotine*
Dibenz[*a,h*]acridine*	N-Nitrosonanabasine*
Dibenz[*a,j*]acridine*	N-Nitrosopiperidine*
Dibenzo[*c,g*]carbazone*	N-Nitrosopyrrolidine*
N-Dibutylnitrosamine*	Phenol
Dichlorostilbene	Polonium-210*
2,3-Dimethylchrysene*	Propene
Dimethylphenol	Pyridine
Ethane	Sulfur dioxide
Ethanol	Toluene
Ethylphenol	Vinyl acetate
Fluoranthene	

smoking. Between 1930 and 1977, the age-adjusted rate of lung cancer deaths among United States males increased about 15-fold (Figure 7 in Chapter 1). The rate in 1930, which already represented an increase over earlier decades, was about 5 deaths per year per 100,000 males; by 1977 it was up to nearly

70. For females, the corresponding rates were a little over 1 per 100,000 women per year in 1930, and about 18 in 1977. Total deaths from lung cancer during 1981 are estimated at 105,000 in the United States alone, with 77,000 among males and 28,000 among females.[17]

Not all of this increase in deaths from lung cancer has been caused by the carcinogens in tobacco smoke alone. The rate of lung cancer has also increased among nonsmokers, particularly among people living in densely urban and highly industrialized areas. Some of the increase is probably due to forms of air pollution other than tobacco smoke. Nonsmokers are also subjected to tobacco smoke in many situations; the importance of this "involuntary smoking" probably has been underestimated. Indeed, the concentrations of some carcinogens are higher in the smoke that comes from the lighted tip of a cigarette between puffs than in the mainstream smoke inhaled by the smoker. Such sidestream smoke contains, for example, a 50-fold greater concentration of a class of carcinogens known as nitrosamines than does mainstream smoke. In one hour of breathing in a smoke-filled room, a nonsmoker may inhale an amount of nitrosamines equivalent to the amount inhaled after having smoked 15 filter cigarettes. Nevertheless, we estimate that about ¾ of all deaths by lung cancer among United States males are caused by voluntary smoking of cigarettes.[18] The corresponding figure for United States females is just over half of that for males. Of the 420,000 cancer deaths expected in the United States in 1981, about 79,800 or 19 percent will probably result from lung cancer caused directly by cigarette smoke.

Carcinogens in tobacco smoke also contribute to cancers in other organs. Cancer of the larynx causes about 1 percent of all cancer deaths in the United States and it occurs about eight times more frequently in smokers than in nonsmokers. It occurs most frequently in heavy smokers who are also moderate-to-heavy alcohol drinkers. Perhaps eight out of nine cases of this cancer are caused by cigarette smoke or a combination of cigarette smoke and alcohol. Asbestos may also be a contributing factor.

Oral cancers (lip, tongue, mouth, and pharynx) account for about 2 percent of United States cancer deaths. It is three times more common in males than females, and occurs about ten times more frequently in smokers. Cancer of the esophagus accounts for about 2 percent of United States cancer deaths and is particularly prevalent in smokers who are alcohol drinkers; in the United States, the rate is four to five times higher in cigarette smokers. Only about 3 percent of those with esophageal cancer survive for 4 years. Bladder cancer accounts for about 2.5 percent of United States cancer deaths and is two to three times more common in cigarette smokers. Kidney cancer is expected to kill 8100 persons in the United States in 1981. The rate is about 1.5 times higher in smokers. Pipe smokers (12 percent of male smokers) and cigar smokers (20 percent of male smokers) suffer roughly the same elevated mortality rates from cancers of the oral cavity, pharynx, larynx, and esophagus as do cigarette smokers but do not have elevated rates of lung, pancreas, and bladder cancers. There are fewer pipe and cigar smokers than cigarette smokers, and these forms of smoking contribute less to the total cancer problem than does smoking cigarettes.[7]

Although the cancers caused by tobacco smoke are usually attributed directly to its chemical carcinogens, these may not be the only factors. The observation that cigarette smokers suffer from increased susceptibility to respiratory infections led to the discovery that the function of the immune system is impaired in cigarette smokers.[19] Because the immune system may be an important defense against cancer (Chapter 10), it is possible that part of the carcinogenicity of tobacco smoke may be the result of a weakening of immune defenses. Studies also show that the clearance of dust particles from the lungs of cigarette smokers is, on the average, five times slower than in nonsmokers.[20] Thus, minute inhaled particles remain lodged in the lungs of smokers for much longer periods, increasing the effective exposure time to particulate carcinogens in cigarette smoke (e.g., radioactive particles) and to particulate pollutants breathed in from polluted air (e.g., asbestos).

The frequency of deaths from lung cancer increases steadily

with age in nonsmokers, probably because of a cumulative exposure to a variety of environmental carcinogens. The same is true for cigarette smokers, although the rate at each age is many times higher, and their relative risk accelerates sharply with age (Figure 3). Cancer deaths among exsmokers are far less common than among continuing smokers, although higher than among persons who never smoked. After 20 years, exsmokers still have more than twice the rate of lung cancer of those who never smoked, but have only one-seventh the rate of those who have continued to smoke.

The data presented here suggest that in the United States, perhaps up to 25 to 30 percent of all cancer deaths, and much

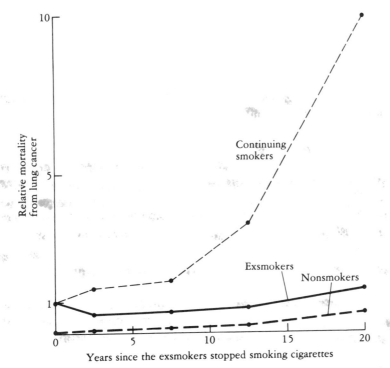

FIGURE 3   Comparison of lung cancer deaths among cigarette smokers, nonsmokers, and exsmokers during a 20-year period that began when the exsmokers stopped smoking. Mortality among new exsmokers is set at 1.[21]

other suffering, derive from the use of tobacco. It is clear that this toll could be much less if people would reduce, or better yet give up, their use of tobacco. A great body of experience indicates that this is no easy task for many smokers. Could it be, for example, that some people inherit a predisposition to becoming addicted to tobacco? In any case, it would seem that an enlightened public health strategy would support vigorous research into the nature of addiction to tobacco and into how to help addicts break the addiction and would work to minimize the recruitment of new addicts, especially among the young. Important research on addiction to tobacco is under way, but whether an effective, comprehensive antismoking strategy can be instituted remains to be seen.

There Are Carcinogens in the Air

The amounts and kinds of chemical carcinogens in the air vary enormously from place to place and from time to time. In general, their concentrations are correlated with urban and industrial air pollution. A few carcinogens are almost always so widespread in urban air that their specific sources are difficult to identify. Asbestos, for example, is used in many manufactured products including automobile brake shoes and thermal and acoustical insulation. Exhausts from motor vehicles are probably the major source of carcinogens in urban air; industrial exhausts are a principal source in highly industrialized regions. Airborne particulates from motor vehicle exhaust contain a variety of organic substances, some of which are direct mutagens and others of which require conversion to an active form. Some of the latter (for example, the well-known precarcinogen benzo[*a*]pyrene) apparently undergo conversion to carcinogens in the air by reacting chemically with other air pollutants (for example, nitrogen dioxide and nitric acid). Thus, it is not surprising that particulate air pollutants collected over such cities as Los Angeles contain a variety of chemicals that are mutagenic for bacteria and also carcinogenic in experimental animals.[22] Presumably these airborne particles are at least in part responsible for the higher rates of lung cancer and possibly other cancers that city dwellers experience.

Numerous other chemicals are released into the atmosphere (sometimes in large amounts) in the form of industrial gases, fumes, smoke, and dusts. How important these are to the total cancer problem remains to be determined, but undoubtedly they do contribute. For example, members of a community in Scotland, who live downwind from a nearby steel foundry from which they received large amounts of polluted air, had a death rate from respiratory cancer about four times higher than persons in comparable communities located in other directions from the foundry.[23] It seems likely that fumes from the foundry are the cause of the increased rate of respiratory cancers downwind. A few other similarly direct associations between industrial air pollution and elevated cancer rates in nearby communities are known, and no doubt many more remain to be recognized.

There Are Carcinogens in Drinking Water

Drinking water was formerly the major route for the spread of infectious diseases, for example, cholera and typhoid fever. These diseases have been virtually eliminated in many parts of the world through modern sanitation practices, particularly the chlorination of municipal water supplies—a mixed blessing, as you will see. The study of drinking water as a vehicle for chemical carcinogens, however, has only just begun, and facts are still few.

One of the most widely distributed carcinogens known to occur in drinking water is asbestos. Its concentration in water supplies in United States cities usually varies from less than 0.1 microgram/liter to more than 200 micrograms/liter.[24] Elevated levels are particularly encountered in drinking water derived from lakes and rivers into which mine tailings are dumped. Lake Superior is a major example of a water supply that is heavily polluted with asbestos fibers by mining industries. This water is piped to millions of people in communities bordering the lake. Because of the known role of airborne asbestos in lung cancer, there is much concern about waterborne asbestos, but as yet we have no clear information about the dangers of ingested asbestos.

Municipal water supplies generally contain very low levels of organic compounds, some of which are known to be carcinogenic in animals (Tables 2 and 3). In total, more than 300 different chemicals have been identified in drinking water. Some of these are converted from noncarcinogens into carcinogens, for example, chloroform and carbon tetrachloride, by routine chlorination in water treatment plants. Other chemicals derive primarily from industrial wastes, for example, carbon disulfide and vinyl chloride. Still others are agricultural chemicals, for example, DDT, heptachlor, and dieldrin, that arrive in runoff from irrigated farms.

Although the amounts of chemical carcinogens in drinking

TABLE 2. Partial list of chemical carcinogens or precarcinogens in the drinking water of several United States cities.[25]

	New Orleans, LA	Miami, FL	Seattle, WA	Philadelphia, PA	Cincinnati, OH	Tucson, AZ	New York, NY	Grand Forks, ND
Benzene	+	+		+	+			
Chloromethyl ether	+							
Vinyl chloride		+			+			
DDT	+				+			
Dieldrin	+	+	+		+			
Hexachlorocyclohexane					+			
Bis(2-chloroethyl) ether	+				+			
Carbon tetrachloride	+	+		+	+		+	+
Chloroform	+	+	+	+	+	+	+	+
Heptachlor	+	+			+	+	+	
Pentachlorobiphenyl					+			
Tetrachlorobiphenyl					+			
Trichlorobiphenyl					+			
Carbon disulfide	+	+			+	+		+

TABLE 3. Chemicals suspected of being carcinogens detected in the drinking water of several United States cities.[25]

	New Orleans, LA	Miami, FL	Seattle, WA	Philadelphia, PA	Cincinnati, OH	Tucson, AZ	New York, NY	Grand Forks, ND
Acetaldehyde	+	+	+	+	+			
Bis(2-chloroisopropyl) ether	+							
Hexachlorobenzene	+							
Tetrachloroethylene	+	+		+	+		+	+
1,4-Dichlorobenzene	+	+		+	+			
Endrin	+				+			
Methyl stearate					+			
Atrazine	+							
Bromodichloromethane	+	+	+	+	+		+	+
Bromoform	+	+		+	+	+	+	
Chlorobenzene	+	+	+	+	+		+	+
Dibromochloromethane	+	+	+	+	+	+	+	+
1,2-Dichloroethane	+	+		+	+			
Hexachloroethane	+	+						
Methylene chloride	+	+	+	+	+		+	+

water are usually extremely low, epidemiological studies in Louisiana, Ohio, and New Jersey suggest that some human cancers are indeed caused by carcinogens in drinking water.[25] A major study of 24 cities with fluoridated water and 22 cities with nonfluoridated water supplies in the United States failed to produce any evidence of a harmful effect of fluoridation.[26]

There Are Carcinogens in Foods

Food and drink (other than water) have long been suspected as sources of cancer-causing agents. For example, an association between drinking alcoholic beverages and cancers of the mouth, pharynx, larynx, and esophagus was recognized more than 50 years ago.[27] More recently, liver and lung cancers have been added to the list. It is not known, however, whether alcohol itself is carcinogenic. Pure alcohol does not cause mutations in bacteria and does not seem to produce cancer in laboratory animals. These observations suggest that some other component of alcoholic beverages may be carcinogenic. Many kinds of alcoholic beverages (beer, whiskey, cider) do contain small amounts of chemical carcinogens known as nitrosamines (see following). Alternatively, alcohol may increase susceptibility to other chemical carcinogens. In one study of men in France, the rate of esophageal cancer was found to go up with increased use of alcohol in conjunction with heavier cigarette smoking. That is, among men who used the equivalent of at least a half-pint of whiskey and 40 or more cigarettes per day, the rate of esophageal cancer was 45 times greater than among men who used the equivalent of at most a quarter-pint of whiskey and no more than 10 cigarettes per day.[28] A study of United States patients with laryngeal cancer showed that the occurrence of this cancer was proportional to the consumption of alcohol: the greater the intake, the more frequent the cancer. The same study also confirmed that cigarette smoking sharply increased the rate of laryngeal cancer and also suggested that dental X rays might also increase the rate of this cancer.[29] Among United States women who both smoked and drank, oral cancers developed several years earlier, on the average, than among women who smoked but did not drink.[29] These and other studies support the idea that alcohol may make cells more susceptible to carcinogens present in tobacco smoke.

One of the earliest suggestions of an association between diet and cancer was the observation that esophageal cancer was more frequent among heavy tea drinkers. In the eighteenth century, tea had become the national drink of Holland, and the frequency of esophageal cancer among the Dutch was uncommonly high.[30] The British may have escaped this presumed carcinogenicity because they add milk to their tea, which may have inactivated the carcinogen(s). Subsequently, the Dutch switched from tea to coffee, and esophageal cancer became rare in Holland. The rate of esophageal cancer is today high in certain areas of Japan where a tea–rice gruel is consumed in large amounts.[31]

These observations are only suggestive and do not *prove* that tea causes esophageal or any other kind of cancer. However, a material extracted from tea (tannin) was repeatedly injected into rats with the result that 26 out of 30 of the animals developed cancers.[32]

Evidence suggests that coffee may be carcinogenic. Caffeine causes mutations in bacteria and causes chromosome damage in mammalian cells grown in culture but apparently does not cause mutations in mammals themselves, probably because it is rapidly detoxified in the body.[33]

In addition to tea, a number of other plants contain carcinogens, but fortunately few of these are part of common human diets. Bracken fern is sometimes eaten by cattle, which subsequently develop bladder cancer. Bracken fern also causes intestinal cancer in laboratory rats and quail and lung cancer in mice. The substance safrole occurs in several spices and is a major component of oil of sassafras and sassafras tea. Safrole was reported in 1960 to cause liver cancer in rats, and its intentional use in the human diet, for example, as a flavoring agent in root beer, was discontinued in the United States.[34]

A number of dietary carcinogens that do not occur naturally in foods are added or are formed at some stage of processing foods. A particularly interesting example are substances called aflatoxins, which are formed in certain foods. AFLATOXINS are a group of poisons secreted by strains of the mold *Aspergillus flavus-oryzae*. The molds readily grow on peanuts, wheat, rice, corn, and other grains when these are stored under humid conditions. Some of the secreted aflatoxins are absorbed into the peanuts or grains and may subsequently be eaten. Attention was drawn to aflatoxins when 100,000 ducks and turkeys on British farms were killed in 1960–1961. The deaths were traced to aflatoxins in a shipment of Brazilian peanut meal.[35] Aflatoxins were soon demonstrated in peanut and grain products of many other countries. About the same time, a major outbreak of liver cancer occurred among hatchery-raised rainbow trout. In many hatcheries, as many as 50 percent of the trout died of liver cancer. The cause was traced to aflatoxins in cottonseed meal, a component of commercial trout food.[36] In subsequent studies, 90 percent of ducks fed a diet containing one-third part peanut meal contaminated with aflatoxins developed liver cancer and 20 percent also developed kidney cancer.[35]

Studies of the carcinogenicity of aflatoxins illustrate an additional important point about dose–response relations for at least some chemical carcinogens. When rats were fed 400 micrograms of aflatoxins over a 5- to 10-day period, 16 percent subsequently developed liver tumors. However, when similar rats were given only 100 micrograms of aflatoxins spread out over 16 months, *all* developed cancer.[37] Thus, aflatoxins are more efficient carcinogens if administered in minute amounts over a long period than when given in larger amounts over much shorter times. The same pattern applies to other carcinogens. To be sure, continuous administration of a large amount of a carcinogen will induce cancers sooner in some of the test animals, but persistent exposure to minute doses will ultimately affect more animals.

The lesson to be learned from the aflatoxin study is that even extremely small amounts of an environmental carcinogen in air, water, or food may not be harmless—or even represent only a very small hazard. Indeed, this study supports the belief that much of human cancer may result from the cumulative effects of long-term exposure to small doses of many carcinogens.

Luckily, humans (like mice) do not appear to be as sensitive to aflatoxins as ducks, chickens, turkeys, rats, trout, and many other animals. Liver cancer is accordingly rare in many parts of the world, including the United States. In some tropical areas, however, liver cancer is the most common cancer among men. Studies in Swaziland and Kenya have shown that high rates of liver cancer are closely correlated with the amounts of aflatoxins ingested with peanuts, a major food in those areas.[38] To eliminate aflatoxins from the human diet will require modifications in harvesting and storage of peanuts, grains, and other foods in which molds can grow. The necessary changes will be difficult, but can be accomplished, and would be a major step in preventing cancer in certain countries.

As mentioned earlier, benzo[a]pyrene is a chemical carcinogen found in tobacco smoke, in motor vehicle exhaust, and in polluted air in general. It also occurs in foods that are smoked or charred during preparation.[39] Smoked mutton and smoked fish, both of which contain benzo[a]pyrene, are common parts of the diet in Iceland; this may be related to the high rates of stomach cancer in this country. The charred surfaces of broiled fish and broiled meat also contain mutagenic substances, including benzo[a]pyrene. In general, the charred surfaces of fish are more mutagenic for bacteria than the surfaces of charcoal-broiled steaks, hamburgers, and roasts. A commercial product known as beef stock, prepared by boiling beef extract down to a paste, also contains many mutagens.[40]

The importance of the artificial sweetener saccharin as a carcinogen has not been resolved. Saccharin does not cause mutations in bacteria. In 8 of 11 studies in which rats were fed diets containing large amounts of saccharin, an excess of bladder cancers appeared.[41] However, with one exception, studies of humans reveal no increase in bladder cancers among regular saccharin users. The exception was the recent finding that among males the regular use of saccharin leads to a 60 percent increase in bladder cancer. No increased risk was found for females in this same study.[42] It may be, however, that saccharin acts only as a promoter of cancer and never as an initiator or complete carcinogen. For example, among rats fed a substance known to initiate bladder cancer, 4 out of 20 developed the cancer. However, when doses of this initiator were followed by feeding with saccharin, all 35 test rats developed bladder cancer.[43] Thus, saccharin may be a promoter, contributing to cancer only when some other chemical is also present in the diet. If so, then people who cannot exclude initiators from their diets—and few of us can—might do well to avoid saccharin.

Another group of chemicals that probably add to the human

cancer problem are the nitrosamines. As with most other carcinogens, it is difficult to determine how much they contribute because humans are usually exposed to so many carcinogens in air, water, and food and from other sources. Nitrosamines form spontaneously when nitrite (NO_2^-) salts are mixed with amines. Amines are generally present in meat and fish proteins and are formed in large amounts when proteins are digested (to amino acids) in the stomach and intestines. The formation within the digestive tract of hundreds of different nitrosamines is thus potentially possible. A few are also found in cigarette smoke. Of 120 nitrosamines tested, most were found to be carcinogenic in animals, some extremely so.[44] There is no conclusive proof that they cause cancer in humans, but no species of experimental animal has been found to be resistant to these carcinogens.

Nitrites that are involved in forming nitrosamines are not naturally present in meat or fish, although they occur in saliva. Most enter our diets through cured fish and meats. The practice of using nitrates (NO_3^-, as opposed to nitrite, NO_2^-) to cure meats and fish extends back to ancient China and India and had become commonplace in Europe by the middle ages. Curing meats with nitrite salts preserves a more natural reddish color and imparts a pleasing taste. Around the turn of the twentieth century, it was discovered that these effects were due to nitrites (NO_2^-), not to nitrates (NO_3^-) as had been thought. The nitrites arise either as traces in nitrate deposits or from the action of bacteria on nitrates. In the mid-1920s, the U.S. Department of Agriculture approved the direct addition of nitrites to nitrate curing mixtures. Today, nitrate–nitrite mixtures are routinely used to cure ham, corned beef, bacon, hot dogs, sausages, salamis, and many other preserved meats. The nitrites preserve the color we have learned to find attractive and also give these products their characteristic flavors. Together the nitrites and nitrates suppress the growth of spoilage bacteria. In particular, they prevent the growth of the bacterium known as *Clostridium botulinum*, which produces the poison botulin responsible for botulism (an often fatal food poisoning). The trend in recent years has been toward eliminating nitrates from some meat products, for example, bacon, hot dogs, and canned meats, with continued use of nitrites only, because they fulfill both purposes: preventing bacterial growth and preserving color.

However, the practice of adding nitrites to meats or fish sets up a potentially dangerous situation: the nitrites may react spontaneously with free amines to form carcinogenic nitrosamines during curing, storage, or digestion of the food. Indeed, one nitrosamine (dimethylnitrosamine) has been found with disturbing frequency in cured meat products.[44,45] Other nitrosamines (nitrosopyrrolidine and dimethylnitrosamine) are formed during frying of bacon;[46] nitrosopyrrolidine has been detected in rather high amounts in sausage products from some but not all firms. Another nitrosamine (nitrosopiperidine) has also been found in sausages of some producers. All four of these nitrosamines, as well as many others, cause cancer in animals. Although there is as yet no firm proof that they cause cancer in humans, it seems unlikely that humans would be the only species resistant to these potent animal carcinogens. There are, in fact, many indications that nitrosamines do cause cancer in humans. For example, volatile nitrosamines found in a kind of salted fish widely consumed in southern China induce tumors in the nasal cavities or the nasopharyngeal region of experimental animals.[47] Nasopharyngeal cancer is also prevalent among southern Chinese, and the implication that nitrosamines may be causative agents is clear.

It is estimated that less than a third of the nitrites in the human diet comes from preserved fish and meats. The remaining two-thirds is formed within our digestive systems by the conversion of dietary nitrate to nitrite in the mouth and stomach. Whether this nitrite is important in forming nitrosamines, and hence in the origin of cancer, is not known. On the other hand, we do know that there are strong correlations in human populations between ingesting nitrates and nitrites and the incidence of stomach cancer.[48] Ingesting nitrites and nitrates almost certainly means some nitrosamines will be formed, and no animal species has been found that is resistant to nitrosamine carcinogenesis. There is a possibility that reducing dietary nitrates and nitrites would prevent some human cancers. Completely eliminating these agents as intentional additives to meats and other foods would require some alternative means of preventing the growth of possibly harmful bacteria; refrigeration comes to mind. Presumably, the cosmetic effects of nitrates and nitrites on the color and taste of cured meats is of less concern than combating cancer.

The foregoing are examples of possible specific chemical carcinogens associated with the human diet. There are others involving pesticides, herbicides, dyes, and other substances present in food as contaminants. For example, fungicides of the captan type are potent mutagens in bacteria and cause chromosome damage in cultured cells of higher organisms.[49] It is not known whether captan fungicides are carcinogenic. Yet ten million pounds of captans are produced yearly, and traces of these poisons are legally permitted in fruits and vegetables sold for human consumption. At the current approved level of contamination in foods, a person could well consume a few milligrams per day—possibly creating a serious cancer risk.

There are also less well-defined situations in which diet appears to play a role in cancer. The incidence of uterine cancer, for example, increases with increasing consumption of fats (Figure 4). Breast cancer is also related to the intake of fats. How consuming fats might lead to breast and uterine cancers is not known. It has been suggested that excessive dietary fats may lead to obesity and consequent overproduction of the female hormone estrone. Although estrone is a natural human estrogen, it is known to be carcinogenic.

The frequencies of colon and rectal cancers are similarly related to the levels of dietary fats.[51] It appears that eating more beef and other meats (and hence more fats) usually means eating fewer vegetables. At least in the case of colon and rectal cancers, cancer may not be caused directly by the carcinogenic effects of the increased meat and fat in the diet, but rather by the loss of some protection afforded by vegetables or grains. One study has even suggested that eating cabbage, Brussels sprouts, and broccoli reduced the incidence of colon and rectal cancers.[52]

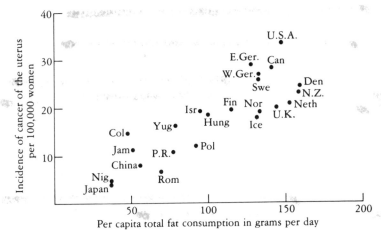

FIGURE 4   Correlation of daily fat consumption with uterine cancer in several countries.[50]

Another possible connection between dietary fat and colon cancer is the fact that bacteria in the colon convert noncarcinogenic bile into carcinogens. Bile is a mixture of complex organic molecules; it is formed in the gall bladder and released into the small intestine, where it aids in digesting fats. The amount of bile released is governed by the amount of dietary fat—the more fat, the more bile. Bile, mixed with grain and/or vegetable fiber and other undigested food, passes rather quickly from the small intestine, which normally contains few bacteria, to the colon, which normally has large populations of various bacteria, some of which might convert bile into carcinogens. High meat–high fat diets may thus result in cancers of the colon or rectum very indirectly. Three observations support this overall hypothesis. First, several potential cancer initiators or promoters are known to be produced by bacteria from bile.[53] Second, populations with higher frequencies of colon cancer also have higher levels of bile in their feces. Third, the feces of a high proportion of normal, healthy persons contain chemicals that cause mutations in bacteria or in chromosomes of mammalian cells growing in culture. The connections between dietary fat and cancers may thus be very complex indeed.

Dietary fiber may also play a role in colon cancer. In people with high-fiber diets, the time that undigested food wastes and bile remain in the intestine is much shortened because fiber accelerates the passage of such materials through the colon. It is thus conceivable that a high-fiber diet reduces the time during which carcinogens could form or act on cells of the colon wall. Some studies on both animals and humans appear to support this idea, but there is still not enough information to support firm conclusions about the importance of dietary fiber in reducing colon cancer.

Although we do not know very much about the problem, it is clear that diet does have profound effects on the incidence of at least some kinds of human cancers. The relationships of diet to cancer have begun to receive intense attention from researchers. A scientific journal devoted to this important topic, *Nutrition and Cancer,* was founded in 1979. Further studies should in time provide the kind of specific information needed to implement effective cancer prevention measures based on modifying our diets.

Some Chemicals in the Workplace Are Carcinogens

Currently about 50,000 chemical substances, not including drugs and food additivies, are in common use in the United States. Many thousands of others are produced but are not commonly encountered by the general population. No more than a few percent of these have been adequately tested for their carcinogenic potential. Some of these inadequately tested chemicals are manufactured and distributed in amounts exceeding hundreds of thousands of pounds per year. The sheer mass of this output poses a potentially severe threat to human populations in general, and in particular to persons whose exposures to such chemicals in the workplace are apt to be great and prolonged. At several points earlier in this book, we described how particular chemical carcinogens were discovered via epidemiological links between particular cancers and certain occupations. Table 4 lists some industrial chemicals associated with cancer. This list is certain to grow as epidemiologists and

TABLE 4. Industrial agents associated with cancer in animals and/or humans.[54] Asterisks denote forms of cancer caused in humans by the agent.

Substance	Occupational Exposure	Kind of Cancer
Asbestos	Asbestos miners; asbestos textile makers; auto brake repairers; cement mixers; construction workers; cutters and layers of water pipes; insulation cord makers; insulators; shipyard workers	Lung*, esophagus*, stomach*, large intestine
Coke-oven emissions	Coke-oven workers	Lung, kidney
3,3'-Dichloro-benzidine	Pigment makers; polyurethane workers	Multiple sites including bladder
4-Dimethyl-aminoazobenzene	Research workers	Liver
4,4'-Methylene-bis(2-chloroaniline)	Elastomer makers; epoxy resin workers; polyurethane foam workers	Liver, lung
α-Naphthylamine	Chemical synthesizers; dye makers; rubber workers	Bladder*
β-Naphthylamine	Research workers	Bladder*
2-Acetylamino-fluorene	Research workers	Bladder, liver
4-Aminodiphenyl	Diphenylamine workers; research workers	Bladder*, liver, breast, colon
4-Nitrobiphenyl	Research workers	Bladder
Benzidine and its salts	Biochemists; dye workers; medical lab workers; organic chemical synthesizers; plastic workers; rubber workers; wood chemists	Liver, ear, intestine, bladder*
β-Propriolactone	Plastic makers; chemists; disinfectant workers	Skin, stomach, liver
Auramine	Dye makers	Bladder*, liver

TABLE 4. (*Continued*)

Substance	Occupational Exposure	Kind of Cancer
Magenta	Dye makers	Bladder*
Chloroprene	Duprene and neoprene makers; rubber makers	Skin
Trichloroethylene	Dry cleaners; drug makers; dye makers; mechanics; printers; shoe makers; soap makers; varnish workers; many others	Liver
Carbon tetrachloride	Firemen; fluorocarbon makers; ink makers; insecticide makers; lacquer makers; rubber workers; wax makers; others	Liver*
Chloroform	Chemists; drug makers; polish makers; solvent workers; silk synthesizers; others	Liver
Acrylonitrile	Acrylic fiber makers; fumigators; plastic product resin makers; textile workers	Colon*, lung*
Ethylene dichloride	Adhesive makers; agricultural workers; Bakelite processors; camphor workers; dry cleaners; furniture finishers; petroleum refinery workers; plastic workers; textile cleaners; others	Stomach, skin, blood vessels, breast, uterus, lung
Mustard gas	Mustard gas workers	Lung*, larynx*
Wood dust	Cabinet makers; carpenters; furniture makers; sawmill workers; wood workers	Nasal cavities and sinuses*
Leather dust	Boot and shoe manufacturers and repairers	Nasal cavities and sinuses*

TABLE 4. (*Continued*)

Substance	Occupational Exposure	Kind of Cancer
Arsenic compounds	Metal industry workers; leather workers; painters; petroleum workers; many others	Lung*, skin*, liver
Chromium and chromates	Electroplaters; gas workers; metal workers; photoengravers; textile workers; welders; others	Lung*, nasal sinuses*
Vinyl chloride	Organic chemical synthesizers; polyvinyl resin makers; rubber workers	Skin, liver*, lung*, brain*, bone
Chloromethyl methyl ether	Organic chemical synthesizers	Lung*
Bis(chloromethyl) ether	Ion-exchange resin makers; lab workers; organic chemical synthesizers; polymer makers	Nose, lung*
Ethyleneimine	Effluent treaters; organic chemical synthesizers; paper makers; textile workers; polyethylene-imine makers	Kidney, liver, lung
N-Nitrosodi-methylamine (di-methylnitrosamine)	Dimethylhydrazine makers; nematocide makers; solvent workers	Kidney, lung, liver
Benzene	Adhesive makers; burnishers; detergent makers; dry battery workers; dye makers; furniture finishers; glue makers; petrochemical workers; putty makers; rubber makers; welders; artificial leather makers; shoe workers; others	Leukemia*

TABLE 4. (*Continued*)

Substance	Occupational Exposure	Kind of Cancer
Soots, tars, oils	Cable layers; coal, gas, coke, petroleum industry workers; coal tar and pitch workers; electrical equipment workers; waterproofers; wharfmen; wood preservers; others	Skin*, scrotum*, lung*, bladder*
Isopropyl oil	Isopropyl alcohol makers	Respiratory tract*, sinus*
Organochloride pesticides	Agricultural workers; insecticide manufacturers	Liver
Polychlorinated biphenyls	Wood preservers; rubber workers; herbicide makers; lacquer makers; paper treaters; many others	Liver
Aniline derivatives	Bromide workers; coal tar workers; disinfectant makers; dye workers; ink workers; leather workers; perfume makers; plastic workers; rocket fuel makers; rubber makers; varnish workers; others	Bladder
Beryllium	Metal workers; miners; nuclear reactor workers; plastic and ceramic workers; many others	Lung*
Iron oxides	Smelters; metalizers; welders; stainless steel makers; steel foundry workers	Respiratory tract*
Lead	Battery workers; brass foundry workers; ceramic makers; glass makers; lubricant makers; painters; plumbers; others	Kidney

TABLE 4. (*Continued*)

Substance	Occupational Exposure	Kind of Cancer
Nickel and compounds	Battery makers; ceramic makers; dyers; foundry workers; paint makers; many others	Lung*, nose*
Selenium and compounds	Copper smelters; glass makers; pesticide makers; plastic workers; rubber makers; textile workers; others	Liver
Cadmium salts	Cadmium industrial workers	Prostate*, lung*
N-Nitroso-morpholine	Rubber and tire makers	Liver

cancer researchers uncover new associations between occupations and cancer and as still more untested chemicals are introduced into the work place. Sadly, the lag of many years will continue between introduction of a new carcinogen and its recognition as an occupational hazard. As a case in point, a higher rate of testicular cancer has recently been detected in metal workers. No specific carcinogen has yet been identified, but presumably it is some form of metal dust. Certain occupations appear to entail a particularly elevated hazard. Rubber workers, for example, suffer an excess of lung, bladder, skin, brain, and lymphatic cancers and leukemias.[55]

In many cases, measures have been taken in the United States to protect workers from known hazards, but in too many situations potentially dangerous exposures continue. Most preventive measures in the United States are relatively recent, such as those instituted under the Occupational Safety and Health Act enacted by Congress in 1970. The newer safety standards have come too late for millions of industrial workers, many of whom will eventually develop cancers caused by years of exposure to one or another carcinogen in the workplace. In most other countries there is little or no control over the manufacture, distribution, export, import, or occupational exposure to known chemical carcinogens. The continued failure to establish such controls over known carcinogens almost certainly dooms entire groups to slow death. When the carcinogen is an ecologically persistent one, the death sentences will not stop at political borders.

There Are Many
Other Sources of Environmental Carcinogens

Dyes are usually organic molecules, and some of them have chemical properties that make them suspect as chemical mutagens or carcinogens. Indeed, aniline dyes derived from coal tars were among the first human chemical carcinogens discovered; they are potent inducers of bladder cancer. The use of organic dyes is widespread, and they occur in many parts of the human environment. The dye Butter Yellow is a powerful inducer of liver cancer in animals. Addition of this dye to food (primarily butter and margarine) was discontinued in the United States many years ago. The use of Red Dye No. 2 in food and drink was banned in 1976 by the Federal Government because of evidence that it caused cancer in laboratory animals. Other, quite similar dyes remain in use, because their carcinogenicities have yet to be specifically established for animals.

Another common use of potentially carcinogenic dyes occurs in the cosmetics industry. In 1975, tests showed that 150 out of 169 commercial hair dyes cause mutations in bacteria. Mutagenic components of such hair dyes need not be eaten but can be absorbed directly through the skin. When rats are treated with hair dyes, mutagens quickly appear in their urine.[56] Two hair-dye components tested were found to cause damage in mammalian chromosomes. These observations strongly suggest that at least some hair dyes may be carcinogenic. One group of individuals regularly exposed to hair dyes in their work are beauticians; a study in Los Angeles county confirmed that beauticians do have about twice the cancer rate as other women.[57]

Medicines are another source of carcinogens.[58] A list of medicines that are known to be carcinogens is given in Table 5. Several are used as anticancer drugs (see Chapter 10). Indeed, most anticancer drugs, of which there are perhaps 30 in general use, are mutagenic and cause cancer in animals. It seems ironic that agents used to kill cancer cells are themselves able to convert normal cells into cancer cells. It is the very killing action of the drug on cancer cells that may lead to damage of a normal cell without killing it; if the damage is of the right type, the normal cell ultimately becomes a cancer cell. Fortunately, the formation of new cancer cells through the

TABLE 5. Medicinal agents that are carcinogens.[59]

Agent	Human Cancer	Animal Cancer
Cyclophosphamide (anticancer drug)	Bladder	Bladder, lung, breast, and others
Diethylstilbestrol (DES) (a synthetic estrogen)	Uterus, vagina	Vagina, uterus, breast, testis, bladder, kidney
Melphalan (anticancer drug)	Leukemia	Lymphosarcoma, lung
N,N-Bis(2-chloroethyl) 2-naphthylamine (used in cancer research)	Bladder	Lung
Oxymetholone (an anabolic steroid)	Liver	Not tested
Isoniazid (an antituberculosis drug)	?	Lung
Phenacetin (an analgesic)	Kidney	Not tested
Phenytoin (an anticonvulsant)	Lymphoreticular cancer	Lymphoreticular cancer
Chloramphenicol (an antibiotic)	Leukemia	Not tested
Coal tar ointments	Skin, stomach, colon, rectum	Many kinds
Arsenic-containing drugs	Skin, lung, liver	None known

action of anticancer drugs is an infrequent event that does not happen in most treated patients. The value of anticancer drugs therefore outweighs by far any potential induction of new cancers.

The drug reserpine, long and extensively used to treat high blood pressure, is reported to be associated with breast cancer in women.[60] Because it is not yet clear that reserpine itself is actually a carcinogen, it is not listed in Table 5. That list will undoubtedly grow because the carcinogenic potential of medicines has only recently begun to receive the attention of researchers.

Some medicines are no longer used because of their carcinogenicity. For example, urethane was formerly used as a sedative but was found to cause lung and other cancers in animals.[61] Thiourea was once used to treat goiter; it causes thyroid, liver, and other cancers in animals.[62]

One of the drugs in Table 5, diethylstilbestrol or DES, is the basis for a particularly tragic story. DES is a synthetic form of the natural female hormone estrogen. During the 1940s and 1950s, DES was shown to cause cancer in various animals.[63] In 1946, DES began to be used to prevent spontaneous abortions, a clinical application of the drug that was shown not to be effective.[64] By 1971, it became clear that some young women whose *mothers* had received DES during pregnancy were developing cancer of the vagina. Young males whose mothers were similarly treated with DES sometimes show abnormalities in their reproductive organs. Fortunately, the frequency of highly malignant vaginal cancer is quite low among the young women who were exposed to DES as early fetuses. This medical episode emphasizes the difficulties in establishing the potential risks of new drugs—indeed of any new chemical.

It seems reasonable to ask, retrospectively, about the efficacy of DES in preventing spontaneous abortions. An answer comes from a study of 1646 pregnant women of whom 840 received DES during pregnancy and 806 did not. Women treated with DES aborted nearly twice as often as women who received no DES (33 versus 17); the number of deaths of newborns was four times higher (16 versus 4) among women who were treated with DES; premature delivery was also higher by about 50 percent in DES-treated women. Thus, DES not only failed to prevent abortion, it was clearly detrimental. These data were published in the *American Journal of Obstetrics and Gynecology*—in 1953.[64] One might expect that the treatment of pregnant women with DES would have stopped immediately, but not until nearly 20 years later, after reports of vaginal cancer in DES children, did the practice finally end. It is not known how many pregnant women were treated with DES, but the number may be as high as 2 million.

Until recently DES was legally used to fatten livestock, either by adding it to animal feed or by implanting pellets in the animals. The considerable weight the animals gain is an economic boon for meat producers. Some of the animals have traces of DES in their tissues, particularly in their livers. Whether this trace amount of DES poses a threat of human cancer remains a hotly debated issue. DES is still also used as a postcoital contraceptive or "morning after pill."

Estrogen drugs also are currently used to treat troublesome symptoms of menopause, and studies of women so treated indicate that they are at higher risk of developing uterine cancer.[65]

Another potentially serious cancer threat was brought to light in 1976 with the discovery that the substance tris-(2,3-dibromopropyl)phosphate, better known simply as Tris, is a potent mutagen in bacteria and therefore likely to be a carcinogen.[66] Tris is an effective flame retardant much used in childrens' polyester night wear. This chemical made up as much as 10 percent of the weight of the fabric and could easily be absorbed into the body through the skin. Subsequent to 1976, Tris was shown to cause cancer in rats and mice, and its use in garments has been banned in the United States. How much it has already contributed to future cancers among children exposed to it probably will never be known.

For a long time it has been debated whether chemical carcinogens have thresholds. Is there for a given carcinogen a level of exposure below which no cancer is caused? Many chemical carcinogens have been introduced at quite low levels into the human environment. Do they represent significant hazards? It is crucial to know whether such thresholds exist in order to make sensible regulatory decisions. The answers may in some cases have enormous economic implications because to remove the trace amounts of many carcinogens encountered in the workplace, in polluted city air, in drinking water, and in food would require enormous costs and effort.

Any health hazard posed by trace amounts of chemical carcinogens should of course be assessed by the best available scientific methods. This soon becomes extremely expensive; as the quantity of the carcinogen becomes smaller, the number of test animals needed to detect an effect rapidly becomes very large. This and other problems of assessing the effects of low levels of carcinogens are further discussed in Chapter 11. Only two key points are relevant here. First, repeated minute doses of some carcinogens are indeed dangerous, as demonstrated by the example of aflatoxins. Second, it is crucial to remember that the effects of carcinogens are not independent of one another but are usually additive. Daily exposure to a trace amount of one single carcinogen might be unimportant, but daily exposure to trace amounts of a dozen or 100 different carcinogens in food, water, air, clothing, and medicines might have the same effect as a single genuinely dangerous exposure to any given carcinogen.

Are Arterial Diseases
(Heart Disease and Stroke) Related to Cancer?

Research has brought to light the possibility that coronary artery disease (heart attacks) and cerebral artery disease (stroke) may in fact be the result of the growth of benign tumors.[67] Stroke (cerebral artery disease) and coronary heart disease both result from blockages of arteries by so-called atherosclerotic plaques. These grow on the walls of the arteries and bulge into the arterial channel, reducing the flow of blood below minimum tolerable levels. Each plaque appears to start from a single smooth muscle cell (smooth muscle cells are normal parts of arterial walls) that has lost the capacity to regulate its cell cycle. If it proves to be correct that each plaque is a small tumor of smooth muscle cells, then most stroke and heart disease could be viewed as tumors. An important implication is that stroke and heart disease may be caused by some of the same agents that cause cancer. Indeed, atherosclerotic plaques have been produced in arteries of chickens by chemical carcinogens, for example dimethylbenz[*a*]anthracene.

The crucial points in this chapter are that chemical carcinogens are widespread in our environment and that nearly all such carcinogens so far identified have been put into the environment by some form of human activity. Realizing this, we can begin to see possibilities for solving a major part of the cancer problem through prevention of exposure to chemical carcinogens.

We return to issues of prevention after surveying what is known about the major classes of carcinogens and an overview of treatments for cancer.

8

Radiation and Cancer

HUMANS are all constantly subjected to radiations of many kinds. These include natural radiations such as cosmic rays from outer space, ultraviolet rays from the sun, and emissions from radioactive elements in soils and rocks. We are also exposed to radiations from medical, industrial, and military sources: X rays, microwaves, and decay products of radioactive isotopes.

There is no practical way to shield ourselves from cosmic rays or from radioactivity from the earth. Fortunately doses from such natural sources are generally quite small. Excluding ultraviolet rays—exposure to which is largely voluntary—these inescapable sources account for about half of the total radiation to which an average person is exposed. A major study conducted in Japan suggests that at least some kinds of cancers occur slightly more often in places with high levels of background radiation.[1] It is generally agreed, however, that at most only a small fraction of all cancers are caused by background radiation. The other half of the radiation that an average person is exposed to comes from anthropogenic sources, primarily medical X rays and industrial and military radioactivity. Exposure to such sources, at least in principle, also *can* be voluntarily minimized.

Large doses of X rays, ultraviolet rays, and some kinds of radioactivity are unequivocally carcinogenic, as this chapter will describe. There is as yet no evidence that microwave radiation (from radar scanners and microwave ovens) can cause cancer. In addition to these electromagnetic radiations, an increasing number of persons are being exposed to sound waves of ultra-high frequencies, so-called ultrasound. At intensities typically used in medical diagnosis, ultrasound waves can cause chromosome changes in cultured human cells. This observation prompts concern that ultrasound may not be as innocuous as is generally supposed. It is estimated that by the mid-1980s almost all infants in the United States will be exposed to ultrasound during routine prenatal examinations.[2]

Ultraviolet Light Can Cause Cancer

Ultraviolet light (UV) is the primary cause of skin cancer. The role of sunlight in skin cancer was well known more than 100 years ago. It is most common among people who spend long hours in the sun over a period of many years and among people living at tropical latitudes, where sunlight is most intense. Skin cancer is so common among sailors and farmers that it was sometimes referred to as sailors' disease and farmers' disease. Skin cancer occurs primarily on areas of the body most exposed to the sun, namely, the face, back of the neck, forearms, and the backs of the hands. It is relatively rare in areas we normally cover with clothing; recent increases in skin cancers in these areas is probably due to the increased popularity of sunbathing and tanning lamps. Sunbathing may account for the steady increase in overall skin cancer rates over the years. In Denmark, where careful cancer records have been kept for many decades, the frequency of skin cancer has nearly doubled since 1945.[3]

More than 400,000 new skin cancer cases are diagnosed each year in the United States alone.[4] The vast majority of these cancers are caused by ultraviolet radiation, a few by X rays and radioactivity, some by chemical carcinogens, and some perhaps by viruses. As in chemical carcinogenesis, the latent period between the beginning of exposure to ultraviolet light and the eventual appearance of skin cancer is usually many years.

Because skin cancers are readily detected at an early stage and while still small, they can usually be surgically removed before they have had time to metastasize (Chapter 2). The cure rate for skin cancer is accordingly over 95 percent, although the preliminary estimate is that 6700 people will die of skin cancer in 1981 alone, up slightly from 1980.[4] Most of these deaths are caused by forms of skin cancers called melanomas, which are cancers that originate in pigment cells. Unlike other types of skin cancer, melanomas are often (but not always) highly malignant because they commonly metastasize at a very early stage, well before they are recognized (Figure 1 in Chapter 1). In parallel with the general increase in skin cancer in Europe and North America, the rate of melanoma is doubling every 10 to 17 years.[5] In Connecticut, where particularly careful cancer records have been kept for many years, the rate of melanoma has increased 6-fold in the last 40 years.[6] Melanomas also tend to occur among somewhat younger persons than most other skin cancers, affecting primarily people between the ages of 30 and 50.

As is the case of nonmelanoma skin cancer, melanomas are more common among people who spend more time in the sun or who live in tropical areas. For example, Queensland, Australia's sunshine state, has the highest incidence of melanoma in the world.[7] A study in Sweden has also linked increased melanoma rates with increased exposure to sunshine; in addition, urban populations were found to be at higher risk than rural populations, suggesting perhaps that urban pollution might also contribute to melanoma. Individuals with thicker, more highly pigmented skin (Blacks, Orientals, Indians) are naturally protected against ultraviolet light. Such individuals develop skin cancer, including melanoma, only rarely.

The worldwide incidence of melanoma is gradually increasing, as we have mentioned. Within this overall increase, the incidence also appears to fluctuate in conjunction with the cyclic variations in numbers of sunspots, increasing at a faster rate a few years after each sunspot peak.[6] Peaks in the number of sunspots are accompanied by a temporary depletion of the layer of ozone gas in the earth's upper atmosphere. A molecule of ozone contains three atoms of oxygen (O_3), whereas a molecule of ordinary oxygen gas contains only two (O_2). Unlike ordinary oxygen gas, ozone absorbs ultraviolet waves. Thus the layer of ozone in the stratosphere reduces substantially the amount of carcinogenic ultraviolet that reaches the earth's surface. The cyclic changes in the ozone layer linked to the sunspot cycle are relatively minor yet apparently result in detectable changes in the incidence of skin cancer. The protective ozone layer is more seriously threatened by technological activities on a massive scale. Industrial chemicals such as the chlorofluoromethanes (used as aerosol propellants, industrial cleaners, and refrigerants), some nitrogen fertilizers, carbon tetrachloride (used as a cleaning fluid, in fire extinguishers, and as an industrial solvent), and jet exhausts released into the upper atmosphere are all known to destroy ozone. Tons of these materials are released into the atmosphere each month. A decrease in the ozone layer of a few percent is likely to increase the incidence of UV-induced skin cancers, including malignant melanomas. It is difficult to predict how large this increase might be, and we will probably have to await the outcome of the 20-year global experiment in which we are currently engaged before we will know. If the outcome is unacceptably high, we could always stop releasing these ozone-destroying materials. Because ozone forms from oxygen exposed to UV, the ozone layer may regenerate itself after some decades. The atmospheric damage might thus turn out to be reversible in the long run; deaths due to increased rates of skin cancers will not.

Much is known about how ultraviolet light damages cells but how it causes cancer is not known with certainty. Ultraviolet light is absorbed by DNA and readily induces mutations. Thus the generally accepted hypothesis is that ultraviolet light is a carcinogen because it is a mutagen. It is possible, however, that ultraviolet light may induce cancers indirectly by generating in the skin chemical carcinogens that are the immediate causal agents.

X Rays Can Cause Cancer

X rays were discovered in 1895, and within a few years persons working with X rays were developing cancers. A man employed for several years as a maker of X-ray generating tubes subsequently died when a cancer metastasized from the back of his hand where he habitually projected the X-ray beam to test the tubes he made. By 1908, cancer had been induced in experimental animals exposed to X rays.[8] Since then abundant evidence has accumulated proving that X rays cause cancer and that, as in the case of UV, the risk is proportional to the dose. For example, radiologists and others who were occupationally exposed to X rays also suffered rates of cancer several times higher than the general public.[9] Improvements in the shielding and focusing of X-ray machines and better protection of those working with them has reduced this risk sharply in recent decades. With modern equipment and techniques, the risk is extremely small for doses sustained in the limited use of diagnostic X rays. For each million chest X rays administered to a population, it is estimated that one additional cancer may be induced.[10]

Risk is proportional to dose. Larger doses of X rays, as used in diagnosis or treatment of various diseases, carry larger risks. X rays have been used to treat a wide variety of nonmalignant diseases of the skin, including the fungal diseases ringworm, acne, and certain other benign skin conditions. Most often, the X rays were directed to the head and neck. One consequence of such therapy is a high rate of thyroid cancer in persons irradiated 10 to 30 years earlier. Before the widespread use of medical X rays in the United States, thyroid cancer was rare and occurred almost exclusively in people over 45 years of age (its causes other than radiation remain unknown). Since that time it has expanded steadily into younger age groups and now occurs in people under 20, undoubtedly because of medical exposures to X rays.[11] In Israel several decades ago, X irradiation was a common treatment for ringworm of the scalp; Israel currently has the highest rate of thyroid cancer in the world.[11] In Denmark, X-ray therapy for nonmalignant diseases has never been used among children; Denmark has one of the lowest thyroid cancer rates.[11] X-ray therapy for skin conditions is still tragically widespread; many dermatologists in the United States continue to use X-ray therapy for acne.

X rays also have been used to treat children with enlarged thymus glands. As adults, these patients experience rates of thyroid cancer some 80-fold higher than the general population.[12] It is perhaps of some consolation that thyroid cancers are less malignant than most cancers, and the 5-year survival rate is high.[4]

Among women given high doses of X rays to treat tuberculosis, the rate of breast cancer is estimated to be higher than that of the general population by a factor of about 10.[12] Again, the rate is directly proportional to dose. Women whose ovaries were X irradiated to treat abnormal menstrual bleeding subsequently experience higher rates of leukemia and cancer of pelvic organs such as the colon, rectum, uterus, ovary, and bladder.[12] Patients treated with X rays to reduce an inflammation of the vertebrae (known as spondylitis) develop leukemia ten times more often than normal. As a final tragic example, children exposed to diagnostic X rays as fetuses *in utero* are known to have higher rates of leukemia and certain other cancers, which may occur as early as the first *two* years of life. The increased risk induced by X rays reaches a peak at age 5 and falls to the more usual general level by age 8.[12]

Clearly, the medical use of X rays has been and will continue to be enormously useful in both diagnosis and treatment; X rays have alleviated much suffering and saved many lives. It is equally clear that X rays have, on occasion, been used imprudently. As a consequence of such misuse, some people have suffered and died needlessly of cancer. The potential benefit of *each* exposure to X rays, including routine chest and dental X rays, should be carefully weighed by the individual considering the exposure against the increased risk of cancer.

Radioactive Elements Can Cause Cancer

A number of radioactive elements emit radiations with biological effects similar to those of X rays. These forms of radiation are known to induce virtually every form of cancer. The carcinogenic effects of radioactive elements were observed even before the nature of radioactivity was fully understood. A form of lung cancer known as "mountain sickness" among nineteenth century miners was subsequently linked to radioactive elements in certain ores. Marie Curie, codiscoverer in 1898 of the radioactive elements polonium and radium, died of an anemia almost certainly induced by exposure to the intensely radioactive ores with which she worked. Radium also causes a form of bone cancer (osteosarcoma) among persons who ingest radium-containing materials for medical treatments or in their occupations. A notable case of radium carcinogenesis in the United States involved a group of perhaps a thousand women, mostly young, employed between 1913 and 1929 at painting luminous numerals on watch dials.[13] The luminous paint they used contained zinc sulfide (a material used in manufacturing modern television screens) as well as traces of radium. It is the radium that makes such paints luminous. These women would lick their brushes with their tongues to keep them sharply pointed, and in doing so, unwittingly ingested quantities of radium, which concentrates in bone, causing osteosarcoma after delays of 3 to 10 years. In the decades following 1913, the frequency of bone cancer among these women increased sharply over that observed in the general population.

The nuclear bombs exploded above Hiroshima and Nagasaki in August, 1945 have also provided grim proof that radioactive substances cause cancer. In subsequent decades, survivors of these bombings suffered increased rates of leukemia and of cancers of the thyroid, breast, lung, stomach, lymphatic system, salivary glands, and uterus.[10]

Similar experiences in the United States occurred between 1951 and 1958 but were made public only in 1977.[14] Significant amounts of "fallout" from 26 nuclear bombs exploded in

Nevada were carried by prevailing winds and subsequently fell on southern Utah. In the affected areas, children born during the period following these nuclear explosions suffered higher rates of leukemia. The incidence of leukemia eventually declined to normal rates among children born after testing was discontinued in 1958. A corresponding increase in the frequency of leukemia was detected among soldiers who took part in military exercises connected with these nuclear explosions.[14] Whether other kinds of cancers were also induced by these nuclear tests may never be known. Very poor records were kept and few of those survive. Moreover, even substantial increases in any one kind of cancer are difficult to detect statistically in relatively small groups (some thousands) of people (see Chapter 11).

A form of radioactive emissions whose carcinogenic significance may have been underestimated until recently comes from so-called alpha-emitters. These include radioactive isotopes of the elements thorium (^{228}Th), radium (^{226}Ra), and lead (^{210}Pb), all of which have half-lives measured in years. Compounds containing these isotopes are present in minute amounts in most soils, from which they are taken up by many plants, including crop plants such as grains, cereals, nuts, and tobacco. The reason alpha-emitters may be important in cancer is that the alpha particles they emit are very energetic. It has been proposed, for example, that alpha-emitters in tobacco smoke become lodged in the lungs, where they may remain for months or even years, constantly irradiating nearby cells.[15]

Radiation Probably Induces Cancers Through Mutations

The effects of radiations on various kinds of cells have been extensively studied. Much has been learned, but the question of how radiation converts a normal cell into a cancerous one has not been completely answered. We do know that at sufficiently high doses, radiation can cause breaks and rearrangements in chromosomes (Figure 1). It was long believed that such gross changes in chromosomes were the basis for the formation of cancer cells; cancer cells often do have many chromosomal abnormalities. It is now known that such abnormalities in cancer cells are not immediately connected with the conversion of a normal cell to a cancer cell but are secondary consequences. Indeed it is now clear that doses of radiation sufficient to cause major, visible chromosome damage to cells are also quickly fatal to most cells. Induction of cancer by ionizing radiations (X rays, alpha particles, etc.) usually occurs at relatively low, certainly sublethal, doses. The key processes in the conversion once again appear to be mutations—alterations of the sequence of nucleotides in a cell's DNA. Recall from Chapter 5 that mutations can profoundly affect a cell's behavior, particularly if they alter genes that normally regulate G1 arrest. These mutations, however profound their effects, are too minute to produce structural changes in chromosomes. As the intensity and dose of radiation to which a cell is exposed is increased, the number of mutations increases. Only if mutations occur in genes crucial for the control of normal cell differentiation and reproduction is a cancer cell created. The chances of such mutations are low. If a person is exposed to larger doses of radiation, progressively more cells suffer progressively more mutations and the chances of forming a cancer cell are increased.

At still higher doses, visible chromosome damage begins. Some cancer cells may be induced at such doses if part of one chromosome is broken off and joined to another chromosome. Thus a cancer cell when first formed may show no chromosome damage (the damage is confined to one or more genes), or it may show a small, specific chromosome change—not gross chromosome damage. Subsequently, through the course of many cell divisions, the descendants of the original cancer cell may undergo more drastic changes in the number and form of their chromosomes. This is the reason cancer cells often have grossly abnormal chromosomes. How these changes come about in cancer cells and what they mean are not known, but they are clearly secondary—developing as a result of cancer—not a cause. At very high doses, radiation induces direct and drastic chromosome damage, which is often rapidly lethal to the cell.

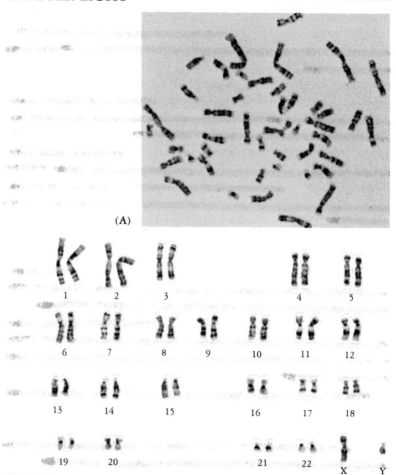

(A)

FIGURE 1   Chromosome complements of normal and abnormal human cells. The banded appearance of the chromosomes was produced by a special staining technique; the two chromosomes in each pair display unique and identical patterns of bands that are used to identify and match them. (Compare with Figure 7 in Chapter 3.) (A) Chromosomes from a normal white blood cell of a male. (B) Chromosomes from a leukemic white blood cell of a woman with chronic myelogenous leukemia. Note that one of the chromosomes in pair 22 and one of the chromosomes in pair 9 are abnormal (arrows). These abnormalities result from a permanent transfer of part of a chromosome 22 to a chromosome 9, and are characteristic of leukemic cells in patients with chronic myelogenous leukemia. Although it cannot be proven that these *particular* chromosomal abnormalities were caused by radiation, changes of this general type are commonly caused by X rays, radioactive substances, and cosmic rays.[16]

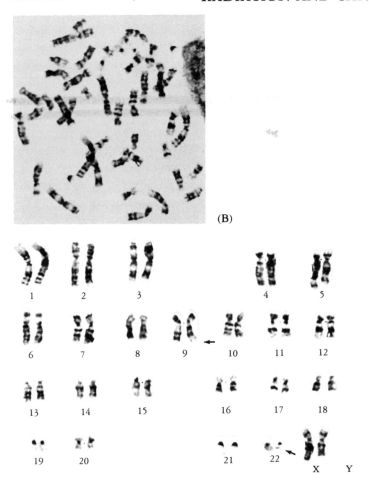

(B)

Thus radiation probably is carcinogenic primarily through the induction of point mutations. In a population of cells exposed to a reasonably low level of radiation, most cells will escape visible chromosome damage but a few will suffer invisible point mutations. A single point mutation in a critical control gene may be adequate to convert the cell into a cancer cell.

Is There a Safe Level of Radiation?

One of the most pressing questions in cancer research is whether there is a level of radiation below which cancer is not induced. That is, is there a safe threshold level of radiation? The question is very important for public health planners and policy makers. It is also a difficult one to answer because at progressively lower doses, the frequency of radiation-induced cancer decreases. At very low doses, the cancer rate cannot in practice be distinguished from the cancer rate in people not exposed to radiation. The problem is that cancer rates can only be determined statistically, and at very low rates small differences become impossible to detect even in very large populations (see Chapter 11). For example, in the period between 1959 and 1977, there were 6 deaths from leukemia among 146 deaths from all causes among former nuclear workers at the naval shipyard in Portsmouth, New Hampshire, where nuclear submarines are repaired and refueled.[17] From the rate of leukemia among all white males in the United States, 1 death from leukemia would have been expected among these workers instead of 6. Do the additional 5 leukemia deaths represent a coincidence or a real increase in leukemia? Although the leukemia rate appears to be increased by 6-fold in these workers, one cannot be certain without more data—more deaths. But

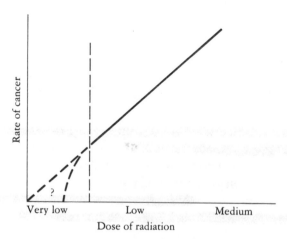

FIGURE 2 The threshold question. The vertical dashed line indicates a dose of radiation so small that responses can be detected only by tests now considered too costly to conduct. The crucial issue is whether there is a dose of radiation below which cancer is not induced.

even small, undetectable increases in cancer rates, if real, can still mean thousands of additional cancer deaths when extrapolated to a national population.

One way out of this dilemma is to use the measurable increases in cancer rates caused by high doses of radiation to estimate how much of an increase in cancer might be caused at low doses (Figure 2). For example, if a given dose of radiation causes a 20 percent increase in cancer, then 1/100 of that dose might be expected to cause an increase of 0.2 percent. The current controversy over setting standards for exposure centers on whether this extrapolation is valid. Some experts argue that the extrapolation doesn't hold and that very low levels of radiation cause no cancer. Most experts believe that very low doses do carry a risk.[18] At the least, they argue, common sense dictates that very low levels of radiation be considered a risk until it can be proved otherwise. Given the enormous costs of evaluating the effects of very low levels of radiation, even in laboratory animals (see Chapter 11), this controversy may not be empirically resolvable in the near future.

9

Viruses and Cancer

VIRUSES cause many kinds of diseases in many kinds of organisms. Virtually every form of life—bacteria and other microorganisms, plants, and animals—is infected by one or another virus. Cold sores, colds, influenza, hepatitis, polio, measles, and mumps are among the more familiar human diseases that viruses cause. One of the first cancer-causing, or ONCOGENIC (*onco,* tumor; *genic,* forming), viruses was recognized some 70 years ago, not in humans, but as the cause of a leukemia in chickens.[1] More than 100 different oncogenic viruses have been isolated since then, and future research will undoubtedly uncover many more.

Most disease-causing viruses affect only a small range of host species and usually only a few kinds of tissues in each host. Oncogenic viruses are generally typical in this respect. A virus that causes leukemia in cats, for example, will not do so in monkeys; a virus that is oncogenic in mice can be injected into rats without effect. Unlike most disease-causing viruses, oncogenic viruses do not ordinarily kill the cells they invade but instead cause permanent genetic changes that result in cancer. The ways in which these changes may occur and their consequences are described later in this chapter.

An assertion that one or another disease-causing microbe—

bacterium, fungus, protozoan, or virus—causes a particular disease must be supported by four kinds of experimental evidence (Figure 1): (1) The suspected pathogen must be found in the diseased tissue and must always be associated with the disease in question. (2) The suspected pathogen must be isolated from the diseased animal and cultured in the laboratory. (3) A laboratory-grown culture of the suspected pathogen must cause the disease when introduced into healthy host animals. (4) Pathogens isolated from diseased hosts produced in Step 3 must be identical with those isolated in Steps 1 and 2.[2]

These criteria are satisfied for the hundred or so viruses that cause a variety of cancers in many kinds of animals, including mammals and primates. This kind of direct and unequivocal proof that viruses cause cancers in humans is *not* in hand, although a number of studies strongly implicate viruses in at least some kinds of human cancers. The difficulty arises in Steps 3 and 4: these experiments would be technically simple but are out of the question because they might be fatal for the human subjects. There are many less direct, less rigorous ways to study the role of viruses in human cancers, and these are described at the end of this chapter. That section, as well as those that precede it, is built upon an understanding of the biology of viruses—to which we now turn.[3]

Viruses Are Intracellular Parasites

Viruses are not cells but rather are parasites that invade cells and are unable to function outside a suitable host cell. Viruses are small, visible only using electron microscopes; so small that many hundreds or thousands of individual virus particles may occupy a single host cell or its nucleus (Figure 2). Thus a cell is many thousands of times larger than a virus. Each virus particle consists of one or a few nucleic acid molecules tightly coiled and wound into a compact mass that is surrounded by a protein coat. Some kinds of viruses also have an additional, outer envelope that surrounds the protein coat. The nucleic acids of virus particles may be either DNA or RNA and rarely contain more than 100 genes. Some oncogenic viruses contain

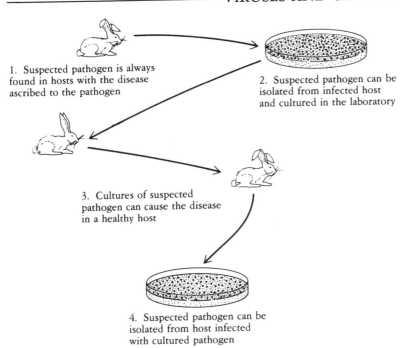

1. Suspected pathogen is always found in hosts with the disease ascribed to the pathogen

2. Suspected pathogen can be isolated from infected host and cultured in the laboratory

3. Cultures of suspected pathogen can cause the disease in a healthy host

4. Suspected pathogen can be isolated from host infected with cultured pathogen

FIGURE 1 The four kinds of evidence needed to establish that a particular pathogen causes a disease.

as few as 4 or 5 genes. Whatever their number, viral genes code for proteins required for the virus to invade its host and to reproduce. Cells, by contrast, have chromosomes that always contain DNA as the genetic material. A cell's chromosomes might each contain thousands of genes—genes that code for proteins that carry out most of a cell's activities. Even the simplest bacterial cell contains about 2000 genes. A human cell probably contains between 50,000 and 100,000 genes.

Virus particles have neither cytoplasm nor organelles and lack most of the macromolecules required for the activities of life. In the form in which they exist outside of cells, virus particles are therefore inert and show none of the properties we associate with living systems. Because its protein coat (and outer membrane, if present) protects the chromosome within,

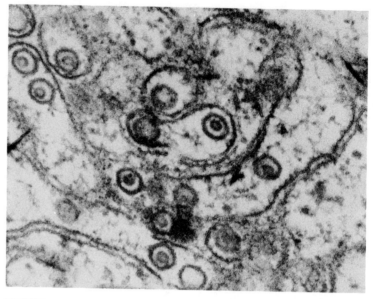

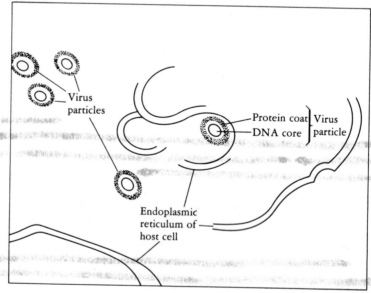

FIGURE 2   Electron micrograph of particles of herpes simplex I virus, a DNA virus that causes cankers and cold sores in humans. These virus particles are forming in the cytoplasm of a host cell.[4]

a virus is well adapted to exist in a dormant state outside of a host cell. Many viruses can remain dormant for very long periods—sometimes years—and survive.

Described in most basic terms, a dormant virus resembles a minimal nucleus stripped of the cytoplasm that would otherwise carry out the instructions encoded in the chromosome. Only by invading a host cell can a virus acquire the metabolic machinery essential for its own replication. When a virus does infect a suitable host cell, it converts the host's cytoplasm into a factory dedicated to producing the components for additional virus particles. It is in this sense that viruses are parasites; indeed, they are obligate, intracellular parasites. The parasitism involves the following stages (Figure 3): A dormant virus becomes active only after it invades a host cell. Once inside the cell, the viral chromosome loses its protein coat and the nucleic acid molecule (viral chromosome) may either remain in the cytoplasm or enter the nucleus, depending on the type of virus. The viral chromosome functions in much the same ways as the chromosomes of the cells they parasitize (Chapter 4). Viral chromosomes are transcribed into messenger RNAs that are translated into viral proteins. All this happens according to the same base-pairing rules and the same genetic code described in Chapter 4 (see especially Figure 10 in Chapter 4). Some of these proteins are subunits of the virus' protective protein coat. Other proteins may interfere with the normal functions of the host cell so that all of the host's resources become available to the invading virus. The virus uses energy generated in the host's mitochondria to produce its own proteins on the host's ribosomes, using amino acids provided by the host but specified by the virus' own genetic program. These and other resources from the host are channeled into synthesizing the nucleic acids of the virus' chromosome as well as the proteins of the virus' outer coat. All of this happens rapidly after a virus invades a suitable host cell. Usually within a few hours many new virus particles begin to assemble from the many copies of the viral proteins and viral chromosomes that have been generated within the host by the invader. Viruses do not grow and divide, i.e., do not reproduce, in the way cells do. Instead, mature

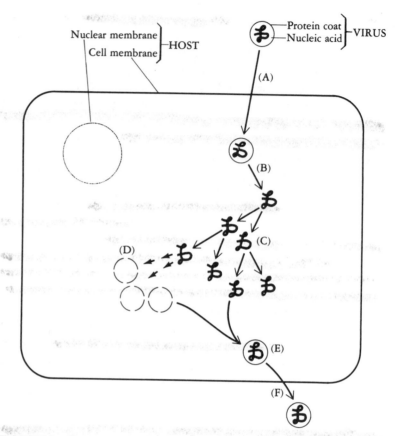

FIGURE 3   Key events in the life history of a virus. (a) A virus particle enters a host cell where (b) the nucleic acid leaves its protein coat. (c) The viral nucleic acid replicates and (d) directs the synthesis of viral coat proteins. New virus particles (e) assemble spontaneously from these components and (f) leave the host cell, completing the life history.

virus particles assemble spontaneously from the viral subunits that accumulate in an infected cell. A single virus particle that infects a host cell may produce many thousands of complete and accurate copies of itself within a matter of hours.

These then are some of the general features of viruses. There are many variations on the basic theme outlined here, variations in virtually every conceivable feature—from the size and chemistry of a virus' chromosome to the effects it exerts on its host. Some of these variations are described in this section; others come up later in this chapter as features of particular cancer-causing viruses.

The presence of many new, active virus particles may cause the host cell to rupture, thereby releasing the newly assembled viruses. Other viruses may be released through the cell's membrane without breaking the cell. These new viruses, in turn, may invade other cells of the same kind, repeating the cycle and producing millions of additional virus particles. In this way, infection of a single cell may spread the virus through a tissue or organism, damaging or killing increasing numbers of cells each time this cycle repeats. Most disease-causing viruses cause diseases in just this way. Each pathogenic (disease-causing) virus invades and damages or kills particular kinds of cells in unique patterns that are clinically distinct. Polio virus, for example, invades and damages several kinds of cells, including those that line the throat and intestines, as well as cells of the tonsils and those of the central nervous system. Most of the tissues damaged by polio virus are those in which G1 arrest is reversible. Lost cells can thus be replaced by renewed cell division among the survivors (Chapter 3). When polio viruses invade and destroy nerve cells, however, the disease becomes irreversible. Sometime in early childhood, all of a person's nerve cells are permanently arrested in the G1 period of the cell cycle. Nerve cells cannot divide to replace nerve cells killed by injury or disease; nor can any other kind of cell divide to form replacement nerve cells. When nerve cells that transmit commands from the brain to a particular muscle are destroyed by polio viruses, for example, that muscle can no longer receive signals to contract: it becomes permanently paralyzed.

Other viruses attack other tissues. Hepatitis viruses damage and kill cells of the liver; the many different kinds of intestinal viruses damage or destroy cells of the intestinal tract; "cold" and influenza viruses damage and destroy cells of the respiratory system; mumps viruses invade cells of salivary glands and sometimes other organs such as the pancreas, ovaries, and testes.

Not all kinds of viruses kill their animal hosts in the short run. Some may remain dormant in the host for long periods, causing no apparent damage. After months, or even years, they may be activated and begin to multiply, soon killing many cells and causing recognizable clinical symptoms. Herpes simplex virus, a common inhabitant of the human skin, is harmless during long periods of dormancy. When activated (usually by ultraviolet light or by some physiological stress to the host organism, such as a common cold), it multiplies, killing localized clusters of cells, forming lesions we call cold sores or fever blisters and canker sores. The activating stimuli seem clear in this case, but the general phenomenon is not well understood for all dormant viruses.

Other viruses are even more prudent parasites. These become active immediately upon entering a host cell but permit the host to survive for long periods, all the while producing new virus particles. The new particles leave the host cell, not by rupturing it, but by passing through the cell's membrane. Such viruses may establish persistent infections in a host animal, infections that endure to be passed on to a cell's progeny at the next cell division or to other cells by cross-infection.

Animals are constantly invaded by disease-causing microorganisms of many kinds, including viruses, yet not every invading microbe or virus causes a disease. Among humans and other mammals, the immune system protects against many infections, including those by viruses. The immune system consists of antibody-producing cells, white blood cells, and the lymphatic system (see Figure 4 in Chapter 2). Only when a virus or other microbe overwhelms or otherwise escapes the immune defenses can it establish a clinically recognizable infection.

The relation of the immune system to cancer is again considered both later in this chapter and in Chapter 10 in connection with possible therapies for cancer. The next section of this chapter outlines what is known about cancer-causing viruses in nonhuman animals.

Oncogenic Viruses

Cancer-causing viruses are generally referred to as oncogenic viruses, although they could equally well have been named carcinogenic viruses. A feature of oncogenic viruses is, as mentioned earlier, that they may not kill their host cells after infection. Instead, they alter the genetic program of the host cell so that normal controls over reproduction and differentiation are disrupted. The manner in which some viruses can cause such disruptions, i.e., can transform a normal cell into a cancer cell, is considered in a later section of this chapter. Here, we survey some important examples of viruses that are oncogenic in nonhuman animals. This survey is a basis both for the discussion of how oncogenic viruses affect host cells and for the subsequent description of what is known about the role of viruses in human cancers.

Viruses are generally classified according to a few important features, including the nature of their nucleic acids, the geometry of their protein coats (and other coverings if present), and the range of host animals they infect and how each host animal is affected. Table 1 lists a number of oncogenic viruses discussed in the following sections.

ONCOGENIC DNA VIRUSES

Smallpox—once a world-wide scourge but now eradicated—is caused by a non-oncogenic virus that carries its genetic program in DNA. There are many other DNA-containing viruses (DNA viruses): some cause diseases, some do not, and some can cause tumors in one or another host animal. For this and many technical reasons described later, DNA viruses are often used in laboratory studies of how viruses cause tumors. Three groups of DNA viruses are discussed here: the papovaviruses, the adenoviruses, and the herpesviruses.

The Papovaviruses The PAPOVAVIRUSES are medium-sized viruses that multiply in the nuclei of host cells. They commonly infect (and can cause malignant tumors in) a wide range of common mammals: rodents, many kinds of farm animals, and

TABLE 1. Major classes of oncogenic (cancer-causing) viruses.[5]

Class	Chromosome Type	Infects	So Far Proved to Cause Cancer in:
Papovaviruses (includes polyoma, SV-40, BK, JC, papilloma, and others)	DNA	Rodents, opossums, dogs, deer, horses, cattle, sheep, monkeys, humans, and other species	Rodents, rabbits, cattle
Adenoviruses (many kinds)	DNA	Widespread, including many kinds in humans	Rodents
Herpesviruses (many kinds)	DNA	Widespread, including five major kinds in humans	Monkeys, rabbits, guinea pigs, frogs, chickens
B-type viruses (milk virus)	RNA	Rodents, monkeys, humans	Mice
C-type viruses (many)	RNA	Virtually all birds and mammals, including humans	Virtually all laboratory birds and mammals

monkeys. Certain papovaviruses have been found in human cancer tissues, raising the suspicion that they may cause cancer in humans.[6] In some animals forms of skin cancer can also be caused by papovaviruses known as papilloma viruses, but there is little evidence to suggest that viruses play more than a very minor role in skin cancer in humans.[7] Common warts, which are benign skin tumors that occur primarily in children and young adults, are caused by a papilloma virus. These benign tumors almost always disappear spontaneously when left untreated. In certain rare instances, they do develop into cancers (see Chapter 10).

Mouse Polyoma Viruses   The most thoroughly studied papovaviruses are polyoma virus and SV-40. All of the major kinds of cancers can be produced in one or another kind of animal by one or another oncogenic virus. At least a few viruses can cause more than one kind of cancer. A particularly versatile virus was first isolated from a salivary gland tumor in a mouse.[8] It was later found to induce over 20 different kinds of tumors in mice, including tumors of the lungs, kidneys, liver, nervous tissues, blood vessels, skin, bone, and connective tissues. This versatility amply justified the name POLYOMA (many tumors) (Figure 4).

The versatility of the original mouse polyoma virus is striking. When injected into a single mouse, it may cause more than ten different kinds of cancers. In addition, mouse polyoma virus causes cancers of many kinds in many other mammalian hosts, including hamsters, guinea pigs, rabbits, and rats. The

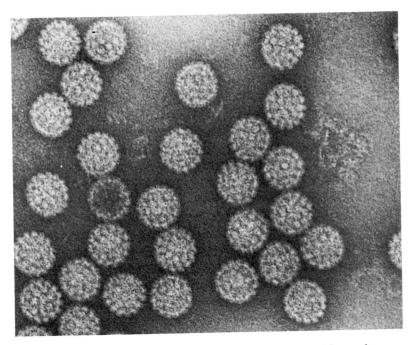

FIGURE 4   A photograph of polyoma viruses taken with an electron microscope. This virus, which is representative of the papova group, causes multiple kinds of cancers in mice. Simian virus 40 (SV-40) is essentially identical in appearance to polyoma virus.[9]

discovery that a single kind of oncogenic virus could cause many different types of cancers, depending upon which organ or tissue it invaded, was important because it confirmed that "cancer" is a family of related diseases, rather than a group of separate diseases. Mouse polyoma virus apparently does not cause cancer in humans and is therefore considered a "safe" virus to use in the experimental study of animal cancer in the laboratory.

SV-40 Virus Another "safe" oncogenic papovavirus is called SV-40, an abbreviation for simian virus 40 (Figure 4). The virus was first discovered in laboratory cultures of kidney cells from monkeys; simian means "ape-like" or "monkey-like." When injected into baby hamsters and into certain types of mice, SV-40 virus induces sarcomas. By contrast with its versatile relative the mouse polyoma virus, SV-40 induces relatively few kinds of cancers when injected in baby hamsters and mice.

Some of the evidence that SV-40 does *not* cause tumors in humans was provided by the inadvertent injection (as a contaminant in polio vaccine) of small amounts of this virus into thousands of people. Two major kinds of vaccines for immunization of humans against polio virus were developed during the 1950s. One of these, the Salk vaccine, contained polio virus particles that were treated so they could not cause the disease but could still stimulate the body to produce protective antibodies. Much of the virus used to make Salk vaccine was grown in and harvested from cultures of monkey kidney cells, cells now known often to be contaminated with SV-40 virus. But SV-40 was discovered only several years *after* the Salk vaccine was introduced; indeed, it was discovered during research to find out if cultured cells used to produce viruses for vaccines might possibly carry other unsuspected viruses.[10] Thus, unknown to those who produced and administered the Salk vaccine during 1958–1961, some thousands of persons were injected with SV-40, along with inactivated polio virus. Although SV-40 efficiently induces tumors in baby hamsters, humans seem not to be infected; there is no evidence that SV-

40-contaminated Salk vaccine caused cancer among any of those injected. Cultured monkey kidney cells are now rarely used to produce viruses commercially, and cultured cells used in making vaccines are now carefully monitored to ensure against contamination with unwanted viruses.

Adenoviruses   Another group of DNA viruses that includes cancer-causing types are called ADENOVIRUSES (*adeno,* gland) and are commonly present in the respiratory tract of humans. More than 30 different adenoviruses have been isolated from human sources. Other adenoviruses have been isolated from birds and from other mammals, including monkeys and cattle. Like the papovaviruses, the adenoviruses multiply in the nuclei of their host cells.

Of the known human adenoviruses, more than a dozen have been proved to cause cancer when injected into young rodents. Some types are more efficiently oncogenic than others, but none has as yet been implicated as a cause of cancer in humans. Many kinds of adenoviruses are generally regarded as human viruses because they are so widespread among human populations, where both the oncogenic and nononcogenic types of adenoviruses are evidently responsible for some respiratory and perhaps gastrointestinal ailments. It indeed seems remarkable that adenoviruses that are commonly present in humans cause only temporary respiratory and intestinal diseases in humans but cause cancers in rodents.[11]

Herpesviruses   The final group of DNA-containing viruses we will describe includes the viruses that cause such common human diseases as chicken pox, cold sores, and infectious mononucleosis. These are the HERPESVIRUSES, which are large viruses that multiply in the nuclei of host cells.[12] Herpesviruses infect most kinds of vertebrates, including humans. Herpesviruses cause cancers in many animals, including frogs, chickens, rodents, and monkeys. The Lucké virus, for example, causes a form of kidney cancer in frogs. A common type of lymphoma in chickens (known as Marek's disease) is caused by another herpesvirus. This latter virus was the first cancer-causing virus that was shown to spread from animal to animal, i.e., to be contagious. Mature virus particles are released through feather follicles and can spread rapidly throughout a flock. In the past, Marek's disease devastated commercial chicken farms, but a highly effective vaccine that prevents the disease is now available.[13] There is no evidence that Marek's virus infects humans.

Herpes Simplex Viruses   Two kinds of herpesviruses that are implicated in human cancer are called herpes simplex Type I and herpes simplex Type II. Infection with herpes simplex I virus is commonplace; it causes cold sores and cankers on the lips and gums. Whether herpes simplex viruses cause human cancer is not known, but they do transform normal human cells in culture into cancer cells, an important observation to which we will return.

Herpes simplex II generally infects human genital areas and causes characteristic sores (herpetic lesions). Because this virus is transmitted during sexual intercourse, herpes simplex II infections are now *the* major venereal disease throughout the world.[14] The disease can be treated symptomatically to reduce its severity, but unlike syphilis and gonorrhea, it is essentially incurable. Like many herpesviruses, herpes simplex II virus can remain in the body in an inactive state for very long times and usually gives rise to recurrences of the disease. Herpes simplex II, as well as other herpesviruses, has been implicated in certain kinds of human cancers.

ONCOGENIC RNA VIRUSES

Like a DNA virus, an RNA virus is an intracellular parasite: a bit of nucleic acid that is enclosed in a protein coat and that lacks the cytoplasmic organelles for carrying out the genetic program coded in the nucleic acid. The nucleic acid is a molecule or molecules of RNA much like the mRNA of cellular organisms (Figure 10 in Chapter 4). RNA viruses usually multiply in the cytoplasm of their host cells[15] (Figure 5). RNA viruses infect a large range of hosts. Most plant viruses, for example, are RNA viruses. RNA viruses are also common

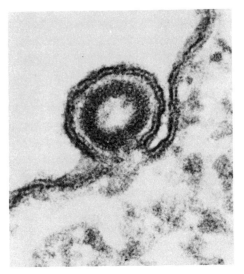
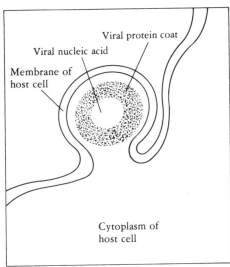

Viral protein coat
Viral nucleic acid
Membrane of host cell
Cytoplasm of host cell

FIGURE 5   An RNA virus that causes leukemia in animals. The virus particle is in the process of budding out of the cell and is acquiring a portion of the cell's membrane.[16]

among insects and other arthropods (e.g., ticks, mites), birds, and mammals. Many infect two or more hosts in nature, one typically an insect or other arthropod, the other a bird or mammal. These so-called arboviruses (arthropod-borne) cause many common diseases, including foot-and-mouth disease of cattle, yellow fever, and Colorado tick fever. Polio, mumps, some kinds of hepatitis, and the many kinds of influenzas that become epidemic from time to time are also caused by RNA viruses.

RNA viruses of one group are known to cause leukemias and lymphomas in their natural hosts, mainly birds and mammals. Another RNA virus causes mammary cancer in mice. These two kinds of RNA oncogenic viruses are described next, beginning with the mouse mammary virus.

The Mouse Mammary Virus   A particularly interesting RNA virus is the Bittner (or B-type) virus named for its discoverer[17]

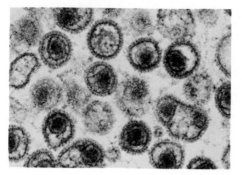
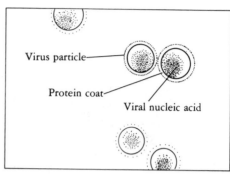

FIGURE 6   Electron micrograph of Bittner viruses from mouse mammary tissue. These viruses cause breast cancer in mice.[18]

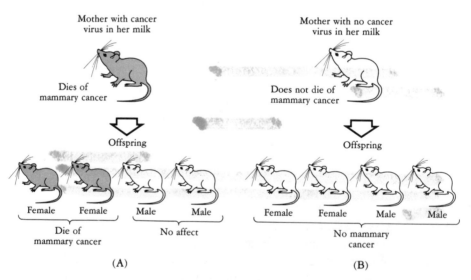

FIGURE 7   (A) A female mouse with mammary cancer virus in her milk transmits the virus to her young as they suckle. The mother eventually dies of mammary cancer and the female offspring die of mammary cancer when they reach adulthood. The males do not develop mammary cancer. (B) The offspring of a female mouse who does not have mammary cancer virus in her milk remain free of the cancer.

(Figure 6). The virus, which causes a form of mammary gland cancer in mice, is transmitted from mother to offspring through the mother's milk. A single drop of milk may contain as many as 50 billion virus particles.

In certain colonies of mice, 95 to 100 percent of all females eventually develop this lethal, virus-induced, mammary cancer; in other colonies only a few percent of the females ever develop the disease (Figure 7). If newborn females from a "low-incidence" colony are suckled by a foster mother from a "high-incidence" colony, most will develop mammary cancers as adults (Figure 8). (Males rarely develop mammary cancers.)

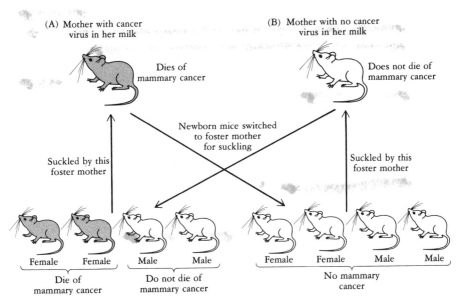

FIGURE 8   (A) When the newborn offspring of a female mouse with mammary cancer virus in her milk are suckled by a foster mother whose milk is free of the virus, these young mice escape mammary cancer. (B) In the reciprocal exchange, when newborn offspring of a female mouse who does *not* have mammary cancer virus are suckled by a female *with* the virus, the young receive the virus, and the female offspring eventually develop mammary cancer. The males do not normally develop mammary cancer even if they receive large amounts of the mammary cancer virus.

Conversely, most newborn females from a high-incidence colony that are suckled by a foster mother from a low-incidence colony escape their fates, so to speak, and remain free of mammary tumors throughout their lives. It is now established that mammary cancer is efficiently transmitted from generation to generation in high-incidence colonies by way of Bittner (RNA) virus in the milk. Low-incidence colonies are free of this virus.[17]

Similar RNA viruses are also found in the milk of other mammals including rats, monkeys, humans; there is no conclusive evidence that they cause cancer, although some experimental findings suggest the possibility.[19]

These milk viruses illustrate an important phenomenon frequently encountered in the development of cancer. The young females that receive the virus through their mother's milk develop cancer only when they reach young adulthood, long after weaning and long after they received the virus. Similarly, in cancers caused by chemicals, radiation, or other viruses, a long period of latency may elapse between the encounter with the cancer-causing agent and the subsequent development of the cancer. These long latencies often obscure the connections between cancers and their causes.

C-Type RNA Viruses The first evidence that viruses can cause cancer was obtained in 1908.[1] A form of fowl leukemia was induced in chickens injected with a crude preparation of an RNA virus obtained from a leukemic chicken. After repeated attempts, leukemia was finally induced in mice by an RNA virus in 1951.[20] A large number of other RNA cancer viruses have been discovered that cause leukemias, lymphomas, or sarcomas in mice, rats, hamsters, chickens, cats, cows, pigs, gibbons, woolly monkeys, baboons, and various other animals. We now know that these RNA cancer viruses, which are called C-TYPE VIRUSES, are widespread among domestic and wild animals.

In many species of animals, RNA cancer viruses are present in a "hidden," inactive form in virtually every cell in any given animal and in virtually all the animals of a species. These hidden viruses are transmitted from parent to offspring directly through the eggs and sperm cells and usually remain inactive for the life of the animal, causing no apparent disease. The transmission of a disease from parent to offspring, whether directly through sperm and egg cells, or indirectly through milk (for example, B-type virus) is called VERTICAL TRANSMISSION. Many oncogenic RNA viruses are transmitted vertically, including hidden viruses.

By means that are not well understood, hidden viruses may be activated by a variety of agents including hormones, radiation, chemical carcinogens, and even other infecting viruses. Once activated, the virus may cause leukemias, lymphomas, or sarcomas: they have never been shown to cause carcinomas (see page 37 for a definition of carcinoma).

When one of these latent viruses is activated, it may behave in one of several ways. First, an activated virus may transform a normal cell into a cancer cell. Often, although not always, the activated virus will also multiply in the resulting cancer cells. Second, an activated virus may multiply in cells of its host without causing a cancer. Multiplying viruses, whether or not they happen to transform a cell, may be continuously released from the cells in which they are produced. Once released in this way, the new virus particles may infect nearby cells in the same animal, possibly transforming them into cancer cells. Alternatively, released viruses may in some cases be transmitted from one animal to another—in saliva, feces, or in other ways. This transmission of a virus from animal to animal, whether or not it results in the spread of cancer, is called HORIZONTAL TRANSMISSION of the virus to distinguish it from vertical or parent-to-offspring transmission. Horizontally transmitted diseases are thus contagious.

RNA viruses that cause cat leukemia and lymphoma (see later), gibbon (ape) leukemia, bovine leukemia, and chicken lymphoma are known to be horizontally transmitted. Situations in which several members of a human family or community develop the same cancer (usually leukemia or lymphoma) suggest that human cancers may be vertically or horizontally transmitted. We return to this important issue later in the chapter.[21]

Feline Leukemia Virus Many domestic cats develop fatal leukemias or lymphomas. The overall combined incidence is typically about 40 cases per 100,000 cats per year.[22] The diseases are most common in younger cats and tend to occur in clusters. For example, in one household, 13 of 37 cats died of leukemia during a 5-year period—a large number compared with the overall rate.[22] This and other observations suggested the possibility of a horizontally transmitted cancer-causing virus. The evidence that this is indeed the case is now overwhelming. The feline leukemia virus has been isolated and studied intensively. It is a C-type RNA virus. As is typical with such viruses, many cats that suffer the disease (about one-third of all cases) do not produce new virus particles because the virus does not multiply in their cells, although the virus is still there and causes the disease. Feline leukemia virus does multiply in two-thirds of cats with disease. Large numbers of viruses are produced by cells that line the mouths and respiratory tracts of such cats, and the virus is spread horizontally from cat to cat through the saliva. The virus invades lymphocytes, converting them into cancer cells. It also invades and multiplies in cells of the mouth and respiratory tract but does not cause cancer in these tissues. Among city populations of cats studied during the early 1970s, about 50 percent were infected with feline leukemia virus.[22] Only relatively few infected cats actually develop cancer. A vaccine has been developed that prevents the infection of cats with feline leukemia virus and thus prevents leukemia and lymphoma.[23] Diligent searches provide no direct evidence that feline leukemia virus can cause any kind of cancer in humans.

Feline leukemia virus is used as a model system for the investigation of human leukemias and lymphomas. The pathological nature of the disease is similar in cats and humans, and the particular cancers are primarily diseases of the young of both species.

Oncogenic Viruses Transform The Host Cells

In contrast to the action of nononcogenic, disease-causing viruses on cells, oncogenic viruses act in a fundamentally different manner when they invade normal cells and convert them to cancer cells. In viral oncogenesis there is no damage in the usual sense from the presence of the virus. Instead, an oncogenic virus disrupts the differentiation of its host cell, interferes with normal regulation of the cell's reproduction, and converts it into a cancer cell. Precisely how an oncogenic virus disrupts normal controls over differentiation and reproduction is obviously a matter of extraordinary importance. Although oncogenic DNA and RNA viruses behave in basically similar ways, there are enough significant differences to justify describing their behaviors separately.

THE ACTION OF ONCOGENIC DNA VIRUSES

A great deal is known about the action of DNA oncogenic viruses, although some critical pieces of information are still missing. Much of what is known comes from studies of virus-infected cells growing in culture, and the following account is based on such studies.

Shortly after a DNA oncogenic virus enters a cell, it loses its protein coat and the viral DNA begins to be copied into messenger RNA molecules (see Figure 10 in Chapter 4). The RNA transcripts are in turn translated into viral proteins. One of the first effects of these viral activities is to stimulate the replication of the cell's chromosomal DNA, which leads to cell division. How the virus achieves this is not known. Infected cells may continue to reproduce for some weeks under the influence of the viral DNA (which itself duplicates within the cell) without producing or releasing new virus particles.

Following the initial period of some weeks of virus-stimulated cell reproduction, almost all of the cells abruptly cease to reproduce and suddenly die. This is known as the CRISIS STAGE of the culture. The few cells in the culture that survive the crisis stage have been permanently transformed by the oncogenic virus and will proliferate indefinitely in culture. Virally transformed cells have been kept in cell culture for over 20 years with no loss of reproductive vigor. In many cases these immortal cells have the properties of cancer cells and indeed will develop into a cancer when implanted into an appropriate animal host. Thus the TRANSFORMATION of cultured normal cells by a DNA oncogenic virus is a model system that has been studied intensively as a means of learning how a DNA virus may cause cancer within an animal. Indeed, the study of viral transformation of normal cells into cells that grow into cancers when injected into a host may eventually reveal how oncogenic viruses work and may also give important insights into the means by which chemicals and radiations cause cancer.

Studies with cultured cells established that a key event in viral transformation of a cell is the integration of one or more copies of the viral nucleic acid into one of the cell's own chromosomes (Figure 9). The effect is that the viral DNA becomes sealed into the host's DNA, becoming a permanent part of the host's genetic makeup. Many copies of the viral DNA may be integrated into the host's chromosome, but the integration of a *single* copy is sufficient to transform the cell. Because the viral DNA is now a permanent part of the host cell's genetic program, it is duplicated and distributed to daughter cells at cell division just as are other cellular genes. Hence, the transformed or cancerous state of the cell is inherited by all of its descendants by cell division.

The integration of the viral chromosome into the host cell's chromosomes also explains how a virus may transform a normal cell into a cancer cell that produces no new viruses. Recall, for example, that no viruses can be detected in about one-third of all cats suffering from virus-induced leukemia. Similarly, in cancer in rodents caused by injected papovaviruses (DNA viruses), virus particles may not be visible in cancer cells. Therefore the failure to detect viruses in cancer cells (as in human leukemia, lymphoma, and sarcoma) does not preclude a viral origin of the human disease.

At least some of the genes carried in the viral DNA continue to be active after the viral DNA is integrated into a cell chromosome. These genes are transcribed into mRNA molecules, which are translated into viral proteins. The virally determined proteins, in turn, are able to change the activities of the infected cell so that it behaves as a transformed (or cancer) cell. Only part of a viral DNA chromosome need be integrated

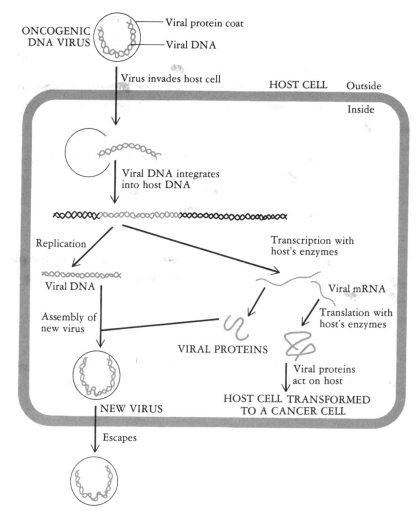

ONCOGENIC DNA VIRUS — Viral protein coat / Viral DNA

Virus invades host cell

HOST CELL   Outside
Inside

Viral DNA integrates into host DNA

Replication

Transcription with host's enzymes

Viral DNA

Viral mRNA

Assembly of new virus

Translation with host's enzymes

VIRAL PROTEINS

Viral proteins act on host

HOST CELL TRANSFORMED TO A CANCER CELL

NEW VIRUS

Escapes

FIGURE 9 Important events in the life of an oncogenic DNA virus.

into a cell's chromosomes in order to transform it. Indeed it appears that only *one* particular gene is needed, and this codes for a *single* protein whose activities bring about transformation.[24]

THE ACTION OF ONCOGENIC RNA VIRUSES

Oncogenic RNA viruses transform cells in essentially the same way that oncogenic DNA viruses do, by becoming integrated into the host's chromosome. The single difference is that the RNA virus must first form a DNA copy of itself; it is the DNA copy that is integrated into the host cell's chromosome.

As Figure 10 shows, the DNA copy is produced by what amounts to a reversal of the process by which an RNA molecule is transcribed from one of the two strands of a DNA duplex. The single-stranded RNA molecule that is the viral chromosome serves as a template for synthesis of a complementary chain of DNA by the usual rules of base pairing (Figure 10 in Chapter 4). The synthesis of this DNA chain requires a special enzyme (called REVERSE TRANSCRIPTASE), which is coded by one of the genes of the viral (RNA) chromosome. The result is a double-stranded helix in which one strand is the original RNA viral chromosome and the other is a new, complementary DNA chain. The RNA strand is then removed by another enzyme, leaving a single-stranded DNA molecule. This DNA molecule then serves as a template for the synthesis of a new, complementary chain of DNA, a step catalyzed by cellular enzymes, producing a DNA duplex. The DNA duplex contains the same genetic information present in the viral RNA chromosome. It is this copied DNA duplex that may be integrated into a cellular chromosome, just as is the DNA molecule of an oncogenic DNA virus (Figure 9). The integrated DNA copy of the viral RNA is transcribed into mRNA molecules (just as DNA of the host cell is transcribed). These RNA copies are translated by the host's cytoplasm into viral proteins, and one or more of these proteins alters the cell's behavior, giving rise to the transformed state of the cell. Further, when the DNA copy is transcribed into RNA, the new RNA molecules are equivalent to new RNA chromosomes that can be assembled into new viral particles.

FIGURE 10 Outline of the steps by which an oncogenic RNA virus ▶ transforms a host cell.

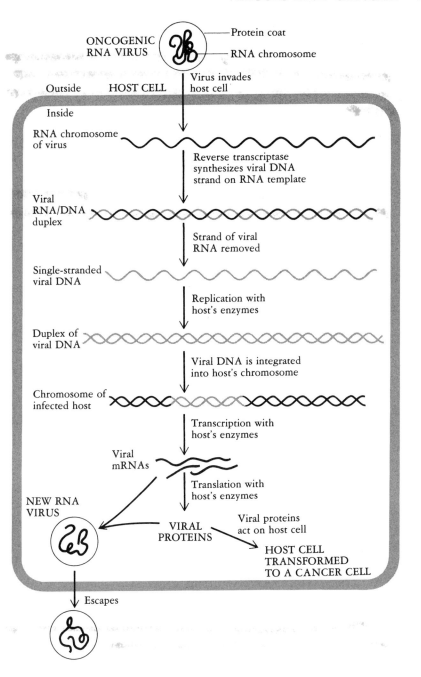

ONCOGENIC
RNA VIRUS

Protein coat

RNA chromosome

Virus invades
host cell

Outside   HOST CELL

Inside

RNA chromosome
of virus

Reverse transcriptase
synthesizes viral DNA
strand on RNA template

Viral
RNA/DNA
duplex

Strand of viral
RNA removed

Single-stranded
viral DNA

Replication with
host's enzymes

Duplex of
viral DNA

Viral DNA is integrated
into host's chromosome

Chromosome of
infected host

Transcription with
host's enzymes

Viral
mRNAs

Translation with
host's enzymes

NEW RNA
VIRUS

VIRAL
PROTEINS

Viral proteins
act on host cell

HOST CELL
TRANSFORMED
TO A CANCER CELL

Escapes

The reverse transcriptase that catalyzes the copying of the original viral RNA into a complementary strand of DNA is an enzyme that apparently is unique to oncogenic RNA viruses. The enzyme does not occur in normal cells, in cells infected with DNA viruses, or in cells infected with non-oncogenic RNA viruses.[25] Thus the presence of RNA transcriptase in cancer cells is believed to reflect either the presence of an oncogenic RNA virus or the presence of an integrated DNA copy of the RNA chromosome of an oncogenic virus. The interpretation can of course be applied even in cases where no virus particles can be found. The latter is an important point: reverse transcriptase has been detected in certain kinds of human cancer cells (see below), and its presence is considered evidence that at least some human cancers may be caused by oncogenic RNA viruses.

Oncogenic Viruses Infect Humans

It is beyond question that some kinds of cancers in animals are caused by viruses; the list of viruses demonstrated to cause cancer in animals continues to grow each year. Because there is no reason to suppose that humans are unique among animals, it seems inevitable that some human cancers will be shown to be caused by viruses. Viruses have indeed been isolated from certain types of human cancer cells, and in some cases these viruses cause cancer in laboratory animals. Such experiments, however, fall short of proving that these viruses are ever the cause of human cancer. Final proof can be obtained only by injecting the virus into healthy human subjects and determining that cancer then develops. Obviously, such an experiment would be unacceptable. Alternatively, suspected oncogenic viruses could be tested on human cells growing in culture. Even if a virus did convert normal human cells into cancer cells in culture, there would remain doubt that the virus would also cause cancer in a living human.

Many C-type RNA viruses have been found that cause leukemia, lymphoma, or sarcoma in animals. Particles resembling C-type viruses have been seen in human cancer cells, but it is not yet known whether they are oncogenic.[26] In monkeys and other animals, it is known that in some cancers caused by C-type viruses no virus is detectable, although the product of a viral gene is usually detectable. The enzyme reverse transcriptase, which is characteristically present in cells containing RNA oncogenic viruses, has been detected in some human leukemia cases, which points to a possible viral cause of some human leukemia.

Similarly, some intriguing findings suggest that a virus may be involved in human breast cancer. The milk of some normal women has been found to contain virus-like particles similar in form to those that cause breast cancer in mice.[27] A virus obtained from breast carcinoma cells of rhesus monkey has been shown to transform normal human/monkey cells in culture. This particular virus has not been seen in human breast cancer cells, but RNA molecules resembling those of the virus isolated from a monkey breast cancer cell have been detected in human breast cancer. Also, reverse transcriptase has been found in human breast cancer cells.[28]

In summary, it seems possible that some human cancers are caused by RNA viruses, but the matter remains unresolved in spite of much work.

The most convincing evidence that some kinds of human cancers are caused by viruses comes from studies of two DNA viruses, both herpesviruses: herpes simplex II virus and Epstein-Barr virus.

HERPES SIMPLEX II VIRUS

Herpes simplex virus is closely linked to carcinoma of the uterine cervix and may be the primary cause of this relatively common form of human cancer. Most women who develop cervical cancer were previously infected with this common sexually transmitted virus. The chances of being infected with herpes simplex II increases with the number of sexual partners. Prostitutes have high rates of incidence of infection with this virus and also high rates of cervical cancer. By contrast, both infection with herpes simplex II and cervical cancer are rare among nuns. Women who marry men whose first wives developed cervical cancer are three to four times more likely to develop this cancer than are women in general. This observation implicates males as the agents by which a possibly oncogenic virus is transmitted from woman to woman.[29] Moreover, cancer of the penis occurs more often among men whose wives have had or subsequently develop cervical cancer.[30] This raises the possibility that cancer of the penis is caused by the same agent that causes cervical carcinoma, that is, herpes simplex II virus. Also, like herpes simplex I, herpes simplex II can transform normal human cells in culture into cancer cells. In a study in England, the average age of diagnosis of cervical cancer fell from 50 years in 1967 to 35 years in 1977, a shift that may be related to earlier initiation of sexual intercourse that has recently become part of our culture. In summary, the case that herpes simplex II virus causes cervical cancer is supported by a variety of circumstantial observations but remains to be proved conclusively.

EPSTEIN-BARR VIRUS

Epstein-Barr virus, or EB virus as it is more often called, is a human herpesvirus that causes a disease known as infectious mononucleosis. This disease is characterized by overproduction of certain types of white blood cells and the consequent enlargement of certain lymph glands, for example, those on the back of the neck. In these respects, infectious mononucleosis resembles a type of lymphoma, but infectious mononucleosis disappears after some weeks. Genuine lymphoma, by contrast, is a progressive disease that, left untreated, eventually kills the affected person. In parts of Africa, EB virus is closely associated with a particular kind of cancer that is known as Burkitt's lymphoma and that is usually confined to children and young adults. Not all individuals infected with EB virus develop Burkitt's lymphoma; indeed, the virus seems to cause cancer only in people also suffering from malaria. One hypothesis is that malaria weakens the victim's immune system, which then allows the EB virus to invade and become oncogenic.[31]

EB virus is also strongly implicated as a cause of a cancer of the nasal cavity and pharynx (nasopharyngeal carcinoma), which is the most common cancer in certain regions of southern

China. Essentially all individuals who develop this cancer were previously infected with EB virus, but only a minority of persons in these regions who are infected with the virus actually develop nasopharyngeal cancer.[31,32] Why the southern Chinese should be particularly susceptible to the carcinogenic effects of EB virus is not known, but there is some evidence that certain dietary practices may create conditions in the nasopharynx that are favorable for the oncogenic action of the virus.

These observations on EB virus point up the complexity of studying viral oncogenesis in human populations. In one population the virus causes a temporary disease, infectious mononucleosis; in a second population the virus appears to cause lymphoma; and in a third population the same virus is apparently involved in the development of nasopharyngeal carcinoma.

The search for viral etiology of human cancer continues at an intense pace. The motivation for this search needs no explanation, but one particular point should be singled out. The identification of a human cancer virus would be the first step toward preventive measures for cancers caused by the virus. It is possible, for example, that a vaccine might ultimately be developed, similar to the vaccines that have been developed against leukemia–lymphoma in cats, against Marek's disease in chickens, and against certain cancers in nonhuman primates (Chapter 10).

Finally, this chapter and the two preceding chapters on chemical- and radiation-induced cancers lead to a partially unified view of the problem of cancer. Much evidence supports the thesis that chemicals and radiation cause cancer by mutating genes whose functions are essential to cell differentiation and regulation of cell reproduction. One may reasonably suppose that an oncogenic virus, rather than causing mutation, interferes with the expression of those cell genes needed for normal differentiation and regulation of cell reproduction. Some experimental evidence does indeed suggest that a protein coded for by a viral gene is the immediate interfering agent.

This chapter completes a survey of the major classes of known carcinogens. In Chapter 10, the focus shifts to the problems of dealing with cancers once they form.

——————————————IO——————————————

Dealing with Cancer

THE preceding three chapters outlined the kinds of agents that cause human cancers: chemicals, radiations, and possibly some viruses. Whatever the causes, the outcomes are similar: normal cells are converted into cancer cells that over-produce, that fail to differentiate or function normally, and that spread to many parts of the body. The conversion seems to involve mutations in genes that ordinarily control cell repro-duction and differentiation.

This chapter surveys the kinds of treatments now available to patients with cancer and to their physicians. For most cancers the prospects for increased cure rates are poor with little con-crete hope for major improvements in the near future. Never-theless, the increase in months and years of life given to cancer patients is already a substantial achievement.

The Effectiveness of Treatment

Without treatment, virtually all cancers are sooner or later fatal, whether directly or indirectly (see Chapter 2). With modern treatments, some cancer patients can be cured; others can be kept alive for many months, even years, without seriously com-promising the quality of their lives. Some cancer patients presently cannot be helped and will die within months of the time their cancers were diagnosed. These differences reflect both the nature of particular cancers and our abilities to treat them.

Cancer of the uterine cervix and nonmelanoma skin cancer can, in many cases, be cured in the sense that former patients remain free of their cancer for the remainders of their lives. Modern treatment of acute childhood leukemia achieves cures in about 60 percent of victims. But for cancers in general, the prospects remain grim. Indeed, it is customary with most kinds of cancers to speak not of cures, but of 5-YEAR SURVIVAL RATES: the proportion of patients who survive for at least 5 years after diagnosis without clinical evidence of their disease. Five-year survival rates for the 15 major cancers that account for 85 percent of all cancers in the United States (excluding nonmelanoma skin cancer) reveal a very mixed picture (Figure 1).

These 5-year survival rates range from only about 1 percent for victims of liver or pancreas cancers to 60 percent or higher for victims of cancers of the breast, uterus, or bladder. Overall, of the estimated 690,000 people who will be newly diagnosed during 1981 as having one of these 15 cancers, some 287,000 (only 42 percent) are likely to survive 5 years.[1] How many of these victims will succumb to their cancers *after* 5 years is not precisely known, but estimates between 12 and 15 percent of persons diagnosed seem reasonable.[2] For example, the 5-year survival rate for breast cancer is about 65 percent but the extended survival rate is less than 50 percent. The 5-year survival rate for prostatic cancer is about 57 percent, but the 10-year survival rate is only about 35 percent.[1,2] Thus, perhaps 30 percent of the people who develop a cancer are ultimately cured, while about 70 percent ultimately succumb to cancer (excluding nonmelanoma skin cancer, for which the occurrence and cure rates are both very high). There has been little or no overall improvement in these figures during the last 30 years or so.

On the other hand, 5-year survival rates are only part of the story. Another important issue is the quality of life for the

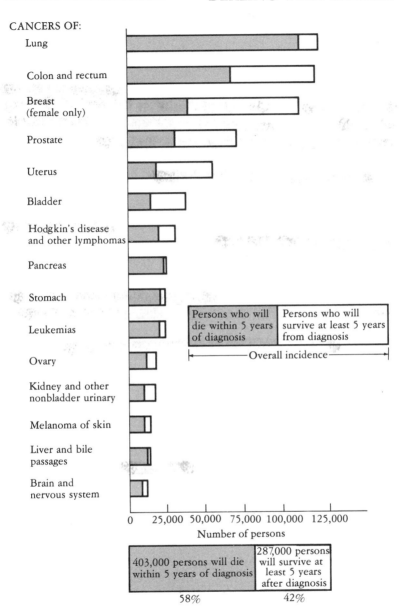

FIGURE 1 Estimated incidence and projected 5-year survival rates for the 15 most common cancers, 1981.[1]

patient being treated. Some of the newer treatments have extended the useful lives of cancer patients by many years, even though cures are not significantly increased.

Three basic strategies underlie the methods now used to eliminate or control cancer. These are (1) to remove the cancer cells by surgery, (2) to kill the cancer cells with lethal doses of radiation, and (3) to inhibit the reproduction of the cancer cells (or kill them) with drugs including hormones. Each strategy has advantages and shortcomings. It is sometimes advantageous to combine two, or even all three, strategies to treat certain kinds of cancers.

All current strategies face the same difficult problem. Most cancers already consist of billions of cells and may have already metastasized to other sites by the time the disease is first discovered. To remove, inhibit, or destroy every last cell of a cancer is extremely difficult and usually impossible with presently available methods. Yet any cell not eliminated by a treatment can, in principle, initiate a new line of the cancer. In attempting to circumvent this problem, researchers are seeking ways to stimulate the patient's own immune system to react against cancer cells. The hope is that, once stimulated, the immune system will continue to operate and eventually destroy every last cancer cell. This immunological approach has not yet yielded a primary therapy,[3] although some researchers remain optimistic. Another recent line of research on which some experts place much hope for improved cancer treatment centers on the substance known as interferon, which is discussed later in connection with the immunological approach to treating cancer. The next three sections outline the three conventional strategies: surgery, radiation therapy, and chemotherapy.

Surgery

If every single cancer cell could be physically removed from a patient's body, a cure could be realized. This, obviously, is the basis for one of the oldest strategies for treating cancer—surgery. Cancer surgery dates back at least to ancient Greek physicians who amputated cancerous breasts, anticipating modern mastectomies.[4] Cancer surgery evolved along with general surgery, becoming both relatively safe and effective only during this century as surgeons adopted germ-free practices, anesthetics, antibiotics, and blood transfusions.

In cases where the cancer can be discovered while still small and localized and before cancer cells have migrated to other tissues, surgery is a very effective therapy. Skin cancers are detected earlier than cancers in other tissues, and skin cancers are effectively treated by surgery. For these reasons, and also because nonmelanoma skin cancers do not readily metastasize, high cure rates for many skin cancers are routinely achieved by surgery. The situation is similar for easily accessible cancers of the cervix of the uterus, and again, cures are frequently realized.

Cancers of internal tissues are less likely to be detected early and are often more difficult to treat surgically. This is so largely because symptoms of internal cancers do not ordinarily appear until the cancer cells number in the billions and, more importantly, have invaded or migrated to other tissues. Lung cancers, for example, usually have already metastasized when they are detected.

In general, the longer a cancer has existed, the greater the chance that cells have separated from the main mass and metastasized to other locations (see Chapter 2). It is usually difficult to predict whether cancer cells have metastasized except by detecting them in lymph nodes or by waiting for displaced cells to generate a new cancer in another tissue.

Refinements in general surgical methods progressively improved the effectiveness of cancer surgery. But the rate of improvement has slowed in recent years, and it is now difficult to imagine any major breakthrough in cancer therapy that involves surgery alone. The fundamental uncertainty of the surgeon's craft—the threat that even a few cancer cells may escape the scalpel—limits the hope that a major surgical advance is even possible. More promising approaches for improving treatments for cancer include combining surgery with other therapies, such as radiation and chemotherapy, and in developing methods that will efficiently detect internal cancers early enough to make combined therapies more effective.

Radiation Treatment

Radiation damages cells and at high doses can kill them (Chapter 8). The intent in using radiation against cancer is to kill a maximum number of cancer cells while killing a minimum number of normal cells. Examples of cancers that are treatable with radiation are certain forms of testicular cancer, Hodgkin's disease (a kind of lymphoma), skin cancer, laryngeal cancer, and some forms of bone cancer. Because radiation can be narrowly directed to highly localized sites, it is frequently effective against cancers that remain well defined. In such situations, it is often possible to kill cancer cells with a minimum of injury to normal cells. Both X rays and radioactive substances, such as cobalt-60, are used in radiation therapy. Once a cancer has metastasized, the problem becomes much more difficult. By the time metastases are large enough to detect, e.g., in X-ray images, they may already have given rise to still another generation of metastases. Locating and irradiating the primary and secondary metastases is difficult and often impossible.

The reasons that cancer cells may be particularly sensitive to radiation relate to the cell cycle. First, cells that reproduce (that progress through the cell cycle) are generally more sensitive to the killing action of radiation than are cells that no longer reproduce (that are arrested in the G1 period). Second, the more rapidly a cell reproduces (the shorter its G1 period), the more liable it is to damage by radiation. Cells engaged in DNA replication and cells in mitosis are particularly sensitive to the killing effects of radiation, although the reasons are not well understood. These properties seem to account for much of the increased sensitivity of cancer cells to radiation. On the other hand, in slow growing cancers the G1 period of the cells is long and the cancer is much less sensitive to radiation and may not be treatable with radiation.

Further, normal cells that reproduce rapidly may be as

sensitive or even more sensitive to therapeutic radiation than slow-growing cancer cells. For example, cells of the bone marrow, which divide relatively rapidly to replace blood cells that die on schedule, are quite sensitive to radiation. In fact, because they reproduce faster than almost any kind of cancer cell, cells of the bone marrow are more sensitive to radiation than most cancer cells. Normal cells of other tissues that turn over rapidly (the lining of the intestinal tract, for example) are also especially sensitive to radiation. When a patient is subjected to a large dose of therapeutic radiation, the intestine and the blood are among the first major tissues to fail, causing radiation sickness, the symptoms of which include anemia, nausea, vomiting, and diarrhea. Cells in hair follicles that form hair also reproduce rapidly and are therefore also particularly sensitive to radiation. Loss of hair is another symptom of radiation injury.

This inherent sensitivity of rapidly dividing cells to radiation damage imposes a practical upper limit to acceptable doses of therapeutic radiation. Current practices of radiation therapy approach the limit, and it seems unlikely that the effective use of radiation can be expanded in any major way. If a technique could be found to increase substantially the sensitivity to radiation of cancer cells only, radiation would become a correspondingly more powerful therapeutic tool.

Even so, two difficulties would remain. One is that *any* therapeutic radiation can be dangerous, exposing patients to the full range of hazards described in Chapter 8, including the risk of inducing new primary cancers. Patients fortunate enough to be helped by radiation therapy may subsequently develop independent cancers in a tissue irradiated during therapy. The other remaining difficulty is that it is almost impossible to eliminate every last cancer cell by radiation therapy alone. A single surviving cancer cell may generate a renewed or a secondary cancer—just as occurs following surgery. For this reason, primary cancers removed surgically may be followed by radiation therapy to destroy cancer cells that may have escaped before or during surgery. This combination of therapies is sometimes more effective than either alone.

The problem of eliminating cancer cells by radiation is also plagued with another complication. Even in a rapidly growing primary cancer or in metastases of the cancer, a fraction of the cancer cells may inexplicably stop reproducing and become arrested in the G1 phase of the cell cycle. Because they remain in G1, these cells remain relatively insensitive to the killing effects of radiation. Such dormant cells are harmless as long as they remain dormant, but they often leave G1 and begin to reproduce after a lapse of months or even years, giving rise to recurrence of the cancer.

Chemotherapy

Chemotherapy is the third major strategy for attempting to eliminate cancer cells. As with radiation therapy, the intention is to kill cancer cells selectively without harming normal cells. In this case, however, drugs, not radiation, are the means employed. A few types of cancers happen to be exquisitely sensitive to certain drugs, and chemotherapy is highly successful in these cases. For example, the drug methotrexate is highly effective in curing a rare cancer known as choriocarcinoma. This form of cancer arises from the placenta during pregnancy and is highly malignant. Chemotherapy with methotrexate achieves cure rates greater than 60 percent for choriocarcinoma. Methotrexate is also used in combination with other drugs to treat leukemia, breast cancer, bone cancer and some others but usually with less effect than in the case of choriocarcinoma.

Methotrexate also illustrates the way in which most anticancer drugs work. Methotrexate prevents the synthesis of DNA during the S phase of the cell cycle. It does so by poisoning enzymes that synthesize the nucleotide building blocks of DNA. Cells affected by the anticancer drug methotrexate are stopped in the S phase, cannot complete the cell cycle, and thus cannot reproduce. More important, a cell that begins to synthesize DNA dies when prevented from completing the S phase. The reason for this is not known, but the overall effect is that in a population of reproducing cells exposed to methotrexate, the cells in the S phase are killed. The drug does not discriminate between normal cells and cancer cells; both are killed if exposed to methotrexate during the S period. Even in a rapidly growing cancer, less than half of the cells will be in the S period at any moment, so the drug must be administered at intervals selected to kill surviving cancer cells as they reach the S period. The drug cannot be given too often, however, because it does kill normal cells. As with radiation therapy, killing normal cells, for example in the bone marrow and in the digestive tract, causes serious side effects such as diarrhea, vomiting, anemia, and loss of hair. Clearly, killing too many normal cells can kill the patient.

Other anticancer drugs such as actinomycin D, cytosine arabinoside, and 5-fluorouracil (5-FU) are similar to methotrexate in their modes of action, side effects, and limitations. Frequently, several anticancer drugs are given in combination. This appears in some cases to increase the killing of cancer cells without increasing the side effects intolerably. Why combinations of drugs work better is not well understood. Which drugs to use and in which combination may be estimated in preliminary experiments in laboratory animals, but the final testing of combinations, doses, and schedules must be done with cancer patients.

Chemotherapeutic drugs are often used in combination with radiation treatment, with surgery, or with both. Again, the reasoning is that if radiation or surgery can remove the bulk of the cancer cells, drugs may be able to kill any remaining cancer cells. In recent years chemotherapy has been widely used in treating many kinds of cancers. The degree to which chemotherapy increases cure rates or extends the useful lives of cancer patients is still debated by cancer therapists.

Chemotherapy for cancer, like radiation therapy, is complicated by the fact that in almost all cancers some cells may somehow become arrested in the G1 period of the cell cycle and thereby escape the killing effect of drugs. Another complication is that cancer cells can become resistant to particular drugs. Such resistance is the result of mutations that occur on the average only once among many millions of cancer cells. Because cancers consist of billions of cells, there is always a reasonable chance that one cell will sustain a mutation that makes it and its descendants resistant to a particular drug. Indeed, because almost all chemotherapeutic drugs are mutagens, they may actually increase the rate at which resistant mutants appear.[5] The outcome of such mutations is that the resistant cells proliferate in spite of the drug. Indeed, the drug may actually favor the resistant mutants by removing competing sensitive cancer cells. Eventually, the resistant mutants will form a drug-resistant cancer. The only recourse is to find another drug that is effective against these resistant cells.

In summary, then, the effectiveness of chemotherapy is limited by three circumstances: (1) that drugs kill both cancer cells and normal cells that are reproducing; (2) that a few cells in each cancer may remain dormant and insensitive to drugs for many months; and (3) that rare, drug-resistant cancer cells may arise by mutation. In spite of these limitations, chemotherapy is effective against some cancers.

Another form of chemotherapy that has been used with some success for certain kinds of cancers is based on hormone treatments or manipulations. Therapy of this sort is effective only if the cancer cells are sensitive to hormones. For example, some breast cancers require female hormones to grow and are actively inhibited by male hormones. Therefore removal of the source of female hormones (the ovaries) and administration of male hormones can retard the progress of some breast cancers. Another important example is prostatic cancer, which frequently can be controlled by administration of female hormones, sometimes in combination with removal of the source of male hormone, the testes.

Some cancer experts believe that our greatest hope is to devise drugs that would selectively destroy only cancer cells without harming normal cells—a sort of magic bullet against cancer. Many thousands of potential chemotherapy drugs have been tested during the past quarter century. Out of this work have come the 30 or so drugs that are currently useful. It seems unlikely that screening an endless series of chemicals for anti-cancer activity will ever yield a powerful and highly selective drug: the haystack is immense and the needle very small, perhaps illusory.

In another approach, researchers have for decades sought biochemical difference(s) that would efficiently distinguish cancer cells from their normal counterparts (see later). A great investment in this direction is justified by two beliefs: first, that specific biochemical differences do exist between cancer and normal cells; second, that understanding such differences may enable researchers to design and synthesize drugs that will affect only cancer cells. The search for exploitable differences has so far failed. In the course of this research, however, our understanding of how cells grow, reproduce, and behave has broadened and deepened. This growing body of knowledge provides a constantly expanding base from which to launch further studies of both normal and cancer cells, and thereby sustains the hope we may someday create the magic bullet.

Early Detection Is Essential

Until a magic bullet is discovered or devised, cancer patients and their physicians must continue to rely on some combination of surgery, radiation therapy, and chemotherapy—strategies that are only moderately effective. Recall that nearly two of three persons discovered to have cancer in 1981 will die of cancer before 1986 ends.[1] Recall, too, that prospects for major improvements in the near future are not good.

The treatments that are now, and will probably for some time continue to be, our main weapons against cancer all work best when the cancer is detected while still small and localized, before metastases have established secondary cancers. Given these facts, every method for detecting cancers early improves a patient's prognosis. For example, only 31 percent of breast cancer patients in whom the cancer spread to four or more lymph nodes survive for 5 years. When fewer than four lymph nodes show evidence of cancer spread, 45 percent survive for 5 years. However, among patients showing no evidence of cancer spread to lymph nodes, 76 percent survive 5 years.[6]

Cancer cells almost always number in the billions *before* they cause the symptoms that then lead to detection. Cancers are therefore usually well established by the time they are detected. An exception noted earlier is skin cancer, which is usually detected before giving rise to clinical symptoms. Major efforts have been made to find simple, quick, and reliable ways of detecting cancer while it is still in the silent growth stage. Palpation (feeling with the fingers) is the oldest of these. For example, 80 percent of all breast cancers are detected by the victims themselves by palpation. But a cancer large enough to palpate has been growing for some time, even when the palpation is done by trained, expert hands that can discover cancer earlier. And only certain tissues and organs can be effectively palpated, for example, breast, thyroid gland, some lymph nodes, and prostate gland.

Other cancers can be detected while they are still asymptomatic by using endoscopes to look inside the stomach or inside the colon. Internal cancers can also often be detected by X-ray examination, but again, for a cancer to be detected with X rays, it must have already grown to hundreds of millions of cells. Sometimes lung cancer is detected by X rays before the cancer has given rise to overt symptoms, but a lung cancer large enough to be visible in an X ray has usually already metastasized. X rays can be used for detecting breast cancers *before* they are large enough to palpate, a procedure called mammography. However breast cells are sufficiently sensitive to the carcinogenic effects of X rays (see Chapter 9) as to make imprudent the use of X rays for routine screening of healthy women less than 50 years old for early, asymptomatic breast cancer.[7] Another method sometimes used for detecting breast cancer is called thermography. The method is based on the fact that breast carcinomas emit more heat than normal breast tissue; this increased heat can be sensed and its location determined by an infrared scanning device.

Many efforts have been made to develop chemical tests for cancer, for example, by using very sensitive assay techniques to detect abnormal levels of enzymes or hormones in blood or urine. This line of research is based on the fact that many kinds of cancer cells do release unusual substances, including enzymes or hormones, into the blood (from which they may also pass into the urine). Although this search offers some promise, it has not yet provided a reliable means of early cancer detection.

The most successful method of early detection yet devised is the so-called Pap smear for detecting cancer of the uterine cervix. The name derives from that of its originator, G. N. Papanicolaou. In this test, cells from the vaginal canal are collected, stained, and examined by microscopy. An expert can reliably tell whether any cancer cells are present. Early detection by the Pap smear is given credit for the steady decline in mortality from uterine cervical cancer.

Cancer of the rectum or colon can also often be detected early by means of a simple test called the occult blood test. Early in its growth, a cancer of the colon or rectum usually causes slight bleeding into the cavity of the colon or rectum, and the traces of blood can be detected in stools by this simple chemical test.

These are examples of efforts toward early detection of cancer, but it is clear that, for the most part, we still lack adequate methods of early detection for all but two or three kinds of cancers.

The American Cancer Society, through its public education program, has stressed that the individual can assist in earlier treatment of cancer by being alert to "seven warning signals."

Change in bowel or bladder habits
A sore that does not heal
Unusual bleeding or discharge
Thickening of lump in breast or elsewhere
Indigestion or difficulty in swallowing
Obvious change in wart or mole
Nagging cough or hoarseness

Prospects for Immunotherapy

Even with early detection, the inherent shortcomings of surgery, radiation therapy, and chemotherapy that were described earlier in this chapter limit what can be done for cancer victims. Researchers have accordingly tried to develop entirely new strategies with which to combat the disease. One of these seeks to enlist the patient's own immune system to destroy cancer cells. This approach—called IMMUNOTHERAPY—has not yet yielded an effective, practical treatment, but it is thought by some experts to offer promise. We explore here the premises and promises of immunotherapy partly because the promise is real, partly because the promise has been unfortunately exaggerated.

The immune system is the main defense against viruses, bacteria, protozoa, fungi, and other disease-causing microbes that invade the body from time to time. Immunological defenses are of two general kinds, both of which involve white blood cells called lymphocytes. These cells are found not only in the blood but make up the bulk of such organs as the spleen, thymus gland, and lymph nodes (see Figure 4 in Chapter 2).

Blood cells called B lymphocytes produce antibodies (a class of special proteins) and secrete them into the blood stream. Each B lymphocyte recognizes and makes antibodies against a different invading microbe, say a certain kind of virus, or a particular species of bacteria. Antibodies play the key role in the destruction of the invader.

Blood cells called T lymphocytes protect against invading microbes more directly. Each T lymphocyte recognizes the surface of a different invading microbe. T lymphocytes, however, bind directly to the invading microbe and only then release a variety of chemicals. Some of these chemicals may kill the invader directly, others may stimulate other defenses, such as phagocytes, which destroy the invader.

B and T lymphocytes defend the body against invading microbes because they can recognize the invaders as abnormal—foreign to the body. These phenomena are often described as the ability of the immune system to distinguish between self (the cells of your body) and nonself (bacteria, viruses, and other invaders). Discrimination between self and nonself usually involves proteins on the surface of the invader that are somehow recognizably different from the proteins normally present in the body. It is these foreign proteins (known as antigens) that stimulate B and T lymphocytes to destroy them, thus protecting the organism from foreign invaders.

Immune responses are a major problem when surgeons

attempt to transplant a tissue or organ from one person to another. The immune system of the recipient recognizes the transplanted cells as foreign (nonself) and destroys them. To prevent the destruction of transplanted cells and the rejection of the transplanted tissue or organ, the patient who is to receive the transplant is continuously given drugs to suppress his or her immune response (immunosuppressive drugs). When the patient's immune system is strongly suppressed, the transplanted tissue or organ may be tolerated long enough to heal into the body. At the same time, however, the immunosuppressed patient is also tolerant of invading microbes and therefore extremely susceptible to infections.

At first glance, it seems plausible that the immune system should provide a measure of protection against cancer. After all, many cancer cells do have unusual surface proteins, and these might well be recognized as being foreign, thereby provoking an immune response that would destroy the cancer cells. Although matters are not nearly so simple, many lines of evidence indicate that the immune system does have something to do with protecting us against cancer.

Two sets of observations seem to support the idea that the immune system is a first line of defense against cancer. One set of observations concerns children who inherit defective immune systems. Children with inherited immunodeficiency diseases (agammaglobulinemia) are commonly recognized at early ages: they are unusually susceptible to infections. An unusual number of these immunodeficient children also suffer from cancer.[8] Similarly, organ transplant patients who receive immunosuppressive drugs develop cancer more often than would otherwise be expected. In both cases, however, nearly all of the "excess" cancer is of a type that involves tissues that normally destroy dead blood cells. Neither of these suggestive observations actually fits with the simple idea that the immune system is an important defense against *all* types of cancers. (Why children with immune deficiency diseases and organ transplant patients should develop only these specific cancers remains unknown.)

Another observation that suggests that the immune system

may be a principal defense against cancer is the extremely rare phenomenon known as "spontaneous regression" of cancer. There are about 200 well-documented cases of patients whose advanced, usually fatal, cancers totally disappeared independently of any recognized treatment.[9] What caused these cancers to disappear is not known. One plausible explanation is that the patients' immune systems were somehow triggered to recognize and destroy the cancer cells. Although plausible, there is no direct evidence to support this explanation. Because it is so rare (only 200 documented instances among millions of cancer patients), spontaneous regression is difficult to study. That is unfortunate because the phenomenon might provide a key to a far more effective way of dealing with cancer.

It is well known that cancer occurs more often among older people. It is also true that the effectiveness of the immune system decreases with advancing age. Some researchers use these data to argue that the immune system provides a defense against cancer. An equally reasonable alternative is that cancer occurs more frequently among the elderly simply because they have been exposed to carcinogens for longer times.

The effectiveness of the immune system is decreased, sometimes severely so, in individuals with advanced cancer, especially patients treated with X rays or chemotherapeutic drugs, both of which are immunosuppressants. Individuals with advanced cancer are, therefore, often especially susceptible to infections by bacteria, viruses, and fungi. Indeed, these infections may be the immediate cause of death, although the ultimate cause is still cancer (see Chapter 2). The weakening of the immune system may also result from some action of the cancer itself. From this observation, it is sometimes argued that the cancer succeeds in growing by somehow weakening the body's major defense against cancer, the immune system. The argument is weak at best.

Many carcinogens do inhibit the immune system. This leads some experts to suggest that at least part of a carcinogen's effectiveness resides in its suppression of the immune system. A few sources of carcinogens, such as tobacco smoke, do impair the immune system substantially. In the case of tobacco smoke, immunosuppression may be important in initiating cancer; in any case it probably accounts for the greater frequency of colds and other respiratory infections among cigarette smokers.[10] However, the degree to which most carcinogens suppress the immune system seems too small to be significant in initiating cancer.

The possibility that the immune system plays a role in eliminating cancer cells is formalized in the so-called immune surveillance theory. According to the theory, cancer cells arise relatively frequently in all normal tissues, but the immune system usually recognizes and destroys these cancer cells. Occasionally, a cancer cell may arise that the immune system does not recognize or recognizes but does not destroy. When the immune system fails in this way, the cancer cell multiplies and produces the disease. The theory is reasonable and consistent with some of what is known about cancer, including many of the observations just cited. Perhaps it is true that cancer cells possess new antigens that evoke a strong response by the immune system so that they are eliminated as they arise. The theory, however, is difficult to test and remains speculative. Indeed, several lines of evidence tend to argue against the immune surveillance theory. For example, strains of mice that for genetic reasons lack thymus glands have severely impaired immune systems. It is in the thymus gland that T lymphocytes mature. According to the immune surveillance theory these thymus-less mice should develop cancer more frequently than normal mice with thymus glands, but they do not.[8]

Recently another kind of cell has been detected in the lymph nodes, spleen, and blood. These cells, which are found in both cancer patients and healthy individuals, are able to recognize and kill cancer cells. These newly discovered lymphocytes (called "natural killer cells") apparently represent a previously unknown branch of the immune system. Natural killer cells appear during development independently of the thymus gland and hence could explain why thymus-less mice are not unusually prone to cancer. Thus, natural killer cells may conceivably recognize and destroy new cancer cells as proposed by the immune surveillance theory.[8] Future research will tell.

Although the role of the immune system in cancer defense

remains poorly understood, some attempts at cancer immunotherapy have been made. These attempts consist of strengthening the immune system by injecting vaccines prepared from bacteria, particularly a bacterium known as BCG (Bacillus Calmette-Guerin) and another called *Corynebacterium parvum*. In a way that is still poorly understood, these vaccines make the immune system more sensitive to all kinds of foreign antigens. In experimental animals injected with BCG or *C. parvum* vaccine, certain kinds of tumors have shrunk and, in a few cases, disappeared. In humans, these vaccines can also slow the growth of certain kinds of tumors, for example, melanomas.[3] However the results have been somewhat inconsistent, and cures have not been achieved.

Mammals produce a natural antiviral agent called interferon. Interferon is a protein produced by white blood cells and certain other body cells, especially in response to infection by viruses. Interferon can inhibit the multiplication of viruses and thereby decrease the severity of, or even prevent, disease. Obviously, the effectiveness of interferon is not complete because we do suffer from viral diseases. Clinical trials in England have shown, however, that colds (caused by an RNA virus) can be prevented by injecting people with large doses of interferon.

In addition to its antiviral action (which could be important in preventing virally caused cancer), interferon also inhibits cell reproduction, although relatively little is known about this facet of interferon. Some evidence suggests that interferon may specifically inhibit the growth of cancer cells.[11] This preliminary evidence has given rise to a great deal of hope that interferon may prove to be a new, effective way of treating cancer patients. Interferon must be obtained from white blood cells and fibroblasts, but the yield is very low. Therefore the supply of interferon is limited and production is quite expensive. The gene for interferon has been introduced by genetic manipulations into bacteria with the hope that the altered bacteria, which can be grown cheaply in large quantities, may provide large amounts of inexpensive interferon. Even if that can be accomplished, years of clinical trials will be needed to assess the effectiveness of interferon.

Finally, antivirus vaccines have been developed that are highly effective in *preventing* certain kinds of virally induced cancers in animals. A type of lymphoma of chickens, known as Marek's disease, is caused by a herpesvirus (Chapter 9). Vaccines prepared from a similar but non-oncogenic herpesvirus completely prevent the lymphoma.[12] Similarly, leukemia in mice and cats can be prevented with vaccines prepared from specific leukemia viruses. A herpesvirus known as herpes saimiri is found in virtually all wild squirrel monkeys (*Saimiri sciureus*) but apparently causes no disease in these animals. This herpesvirus causes a variety of cancers when injected into marmoset monkeys or Capuchin monkeys and causes lymphoma when injected into owl monkeys; most animals die of cancer within a few weeks after an injection. Vaccine prepared from the virus completely protects marmosets from the cancer.[12]

Successes with vaccines that prevent virally caused cancers in animals suggest the possibility of vaccines that would prevent virally induced cancers in humans. The development of vaccines is, however, a long way off. As established in Chapter 9, few viruses have been linked to cancer in humans. The viruses would have to be isolated and identified before the difficult task of developing a vaccine could even begin.[13]

For the present then, immunotherapy remains more promise than practice. Given the inherent limitations of conventional anticancer treatments and the improbability of major improvements in the near term, the prudent strategy is to prevent as much cancer as possible. The next chapter, then, focuses on preventing cancer.

Preventing Cancer

THE human and material resources committed to solving the cancer problem have increased enormously in recent decades. These resources have been overwhelmingly invested in two broad research efforts. One effort has pursued better treatments for cancer patients; the other, better understanding of the disease and its causes.

Research on improving treatments for cancer resulted in the kinds of modern therapies described in Chapter 10: surgery, radiation therapy, and chemotherapy, along with attempts to manipulate the immune system. Measured in terms of complete cures, the fruits of the efforts are small. Although a few relatively rare kinds of cancer can now be cured much more often, the overall cure rate for cancer has not improved significantly over the last 30 years. At the same time, the proportion of deaths resulting from cancer has increased steadily, and cancer annually accounts for over 20 percent of all deaths in the United States. Yet this research effort was not entirely fruitless; with the best of modern treatments many cancer patients do live significantly longer and with more normal lifestyles than was the case a few decades ago.

Investments in basic research, aimed at gaining more understanding about the disease, have in many ways been more fruitful. In recent decades a great deal has been learned about the processes and phenomena outlined in Chapters 2, 3, and 4: how normal cells grow, divide, and differentiate; how carcinogens may affect DNA, mutate crucial control genes, and convert normal cells into cancer cells; how little cancer cells differ from normal cells genetically, biochemically, and structurally; and how cancer cells overwhelm the tissues of the organisms in which they form and grow.

Basic research in a field is often propelled by the conviction that a sufficient understanding of underlying processes and phenomena will eventually yield solutions to practical problems. In this case, the expectation has been that an understanding of the basic molecular, genetic, and physiological properties of normal and cancer cells could ultimately enable us to deal more effectively with cancer. The promise is still largely unfulfilled.

Much has been learned about the nature and causes of the diseases we call cancer. It is certainly clear that the problem is far more complex and refractory than was supposed just a few decades ago. But enough insights have been gained to sustain the conviction that basic research may eventually improve methods for dealing with cancer. So far, however, our practical gains have been small, and the bulk of the cancer problem remains unsolved. One of the most important insights to flow from recent basic research seems to be that merely improving treatments for cancer will not solve the problem—a fundamentally different approach to cancer needs to be pursued.

Much Cancer Can Be Prevented

This third approach to the cancer problem is to *prevent* the disease from developing in the first instance. Prevention is hardly a new approach to cancer, but by comparison with those just discussed, prevention has been largely neglected until very recently. This neglect seems ironic in the light of history. The first occupationally caused cancer (scrotal cancer among chimney sweeps) was recognized 200 years ago.[1] Subsequent experience showed that sweeps could prevent most scrotal cancers merely by bathing more often, taking special care to cleanse themselves of coal soot from the chimneys.

Subsequent experiences in many circumstances established two important principles: that much cancer is induced by agents in the environment and that an environmental carcinogen should be suspected whenever members of some social group (chimney sweeps, watch-dial painters, smokers) sustain, on average, more cancers of a particular kind than the population at large. The action of environmental carcinogens can be recognized in this way precisely *because* the cancers they cause are preventable and are being prevented in the general population *not* exposed to the carcinogen.

These principles have been confirmed dozens of times in the two centuries since Percivall Pott's inference about chimney sweeps. As described in Chapters 6 through 9, a large number of proved and potential carcinogenic agents has by now been identified. Many of these were widely disseminated in the environment or at least in the local environments of workers in certain industries. A few of these environmental carcinogens are now regulated or controlled so that fewer persons are exposed and to smaller doses: some food dyes, some industrial chemicals, some pesticides. But the vast majority of known carcinogens and mutagens remain only partially controlled or even uncontrolled, for example, asbestos, benz[*a*]pyrene and a variety of other polycyclic hydrocarbons, nitrosamines, saccharin, phenacetin, X rays, ultraviolet radiation (sunlight and sunlamps), tobacco smoke, snuff, benzene, aflatoxins, arsenic, lindane and other pesticides, diethylstilbestrol, automotive exhaust, and chloroform.

Some day, a large part of the cancer problem may be solved by policies that prevent the disease by preventing the distribution of carcinogens and mutagens. Such policies can be effective only if based on efficient means for identifying environmental carcinogens and only if administered in socially acceptable ways. Epidemiological data that point to the action of an environmental carcinogen are not alone an adequate basis for preventing cancer. It is not always clear just what it is in the environment that causes the excess cancers sustained by the group of persons being affected. Pinpointing the agent is difficult and is complicated by latency periods of 10 to 30 years, by occupational and social mobility, by differences in life-styles, diets, inherited susceptibilities, and probably by other circumstances of which we are not yet aware. Furthermore, interventions designed to reduce exposure to a suspected carcinogen require still another 10 to 30 years to evaluate by epidemiological methods, clearly an intolerable limitation of these methods, given the human tragedy entailed.

It is therefore necessary to couple epidemiology with laboratory tests for carcinogens, for example, the kinds of tests described in Chapters 6 and 7 and reconsidered in this chapter. These tests are, in a very real sense, another fruit of basic research on the nature and causes of cancer, research that may eventually help to realize the goal of preventing most human cancer. Efforts to develop even more efficient tests for identifying carcinogens are now a major aspect of cancer research.

Different combinations of epidemiology and laboratory tests have yielded lists of confirmed carcinogens, probable carcinogens, and potential carcinogens (see Tables 1 through 5 in Chapter 7). These distinctions are not always easy to make or straightforward to apply, as discussed in the next section of this chapter. Nevertheless, identifying actual and potential carcinogens is a necessary first step toward preventing the cancers they cause. As important as it is to be able to identify carcinogenic agents, doing so will not automatically make it possible to eliminate all human cancer. Cosmic and other kinds of background radiations are, in practical terms, unavoidable, as is a certain amount of sunlight. At a truly inescapable level are the possible mutations that may result from thermal "noise" in the building blocks of replicating DNA, noise that may cause so-called spontaneous mutations (see Figures 11 and 12 in Chapter 4). As we have emphasized, mutations in critical control genes may lead to cancer. The very existence of unavoidable radiations and thermally caused mutations might doom us in principle to some irreducible level of cancer. But these cancers are probably so infrequent compared to preventable cancers caused by agents that can easily be avoided that the toll could be negligible by comparison with current rates. In order to reach the happy state of having to deal with only truly unavoidable cancers, however, we must identify and eliminate the common carcinogens to which we expose ourselves.

Identifying common carcinogens is an essential first step to preventing cancer, but not necessarily a sufficient one. Today we are exposed to large quantities of confirmed but unregulated carcinogens. The case of the carcinogens in tobacco smoke is the prime example of how difficult it can be to put knowledge into practice. Tobacco smoke is probably the most important single source of environmental carcinogens (see Table 1 in Chapter 7), yet commerce in and use of tobacco products remain uncontrolled in most countries. Indeed, the production and sale of tobacco is subsidized and encouraged by policies of the U.S. Department of Agriculture. This agency of our government, charged with restricting harmful chemicals in agricultural products sold in interstate commerce in this country, also promotes the export of tobacco products, and the cancers they cause, to other countries. These policies are continued even in the face of clear evidence that tobacco may be responsible for as much as 30 percent of all cancer deaths in the United States (see Chapter 7). Thus, even when a controllable environmental carcinogen has been unequivocally identified, political and economic considerations have so far blocked measures to control the carcinogen and thereby prevent cancer. Applying the fruits of scientific research is never simple in an industrial democracy because issues invariably arise that are beyond the scope of science alone to resolve.

As established in Chapters 6 through 9, the environmental carcinogens already identified can be grouped into three broad categories: viruses, radiation, and chemicals. Opportunities for preventing cancers caused by these known agents vary from one category to another as well as within categories. Viruses, for example, cause cancers in many kinds of animals. Indeed, every animal species that has been carefully studied is susceptible to at least one kind of oncogenic virus. Humans are almost certainly not exceptional in this regard; several relatively uncommon human cancers even now appear to be virally induced. Cancers caused by oncogenic viruses might be prevented by means similar to those used to prevent many common virus diseases, for example, by vaccines. In fact, effective vaccines have already been developed for some cancers: virus-caused leukemias and lymphomas in cats, chickens, and marmosets (Chapter 10). If particular human cancers do turn out to be caused by oncogenic viruses, it may be possible to develop vaccines that will protect against—prevent—such cancers.

Vaccines against human cancer viruses could presumably be made from viruses harvested from human cells grown in culture. In principle there should be no essential difficulty in adapting the well-developed technology of producing vaccines to this context. However, most viruses infect only one or a few host species (Chapter 9) and ultimately anticancer virus vaccines would presumably have to be tested and standardized in human subjects. That prospect raises unprecedented ethical and technical issues that cloud the promise of this approach to preventing cancer, at least in the immediate future.

The key to preventing radiation-induced cancers is theoretically simpler: avoid radiation. Although putting this advice into practice is not always simple, large numbers of skin cancers, including many cases of highly malignant melanomas, could be prevented by minimizing exposures to the ultraviolet rays of sunlight. In this regard the large-scale production and widespread use of fluorocarbons and other atmospheric pollutants that deplete the protective layer of ozone allow more of the oncogenic power of the sun to reach the surface of the earth and our skins. It is ironic that the current fad of associating a deep tan with good health fosters the habit of prolonged sunbathing and even businesses ("tanning parlors") that rent access to high-intensity ultraviolet lamps.[2] Using X rays and other medical radiation more prudently, decreasing occupational exposure of miners and industrial workers to radioactive substances, and prohibiting the addition of radioactive materials to the general environment are a few of the more obvious steps toward preventing radiation-induced cancers. An important aspect of the debate about the safety of nuclear power plants concerns the carcinogenic effects of the radioactive wastes they produce. For example, there is much argument about so-called safe levels of radiation exposure, below which cancers supposedly are not induced. Measuring the effects of very low levels of radiation is most difficult, and most experts do not accept the idea of a safe level of radiation. Thus, it may be that cancer is induced even at the lowest exposures to radiation but that the frequency of induction is simply proportionally lower. Although the principle of preventing radiation-induced cancers is simple, implementing the principle is not. Again, the barriers to implementing preventive policies are both social and technical.

The same is true for policies that would prevent cancers caused by chemicals in our food, water, air, medicines, clothing, hair dyes, tobacco, and alcoholic beverages. These chemicals together account for a major proportion of all human cancers and thus offer the greatest opportunities for prevention (see Tables 1 through 5 in Chapter 7). Given the rates at which large quantities of new chemicals are being introduced and disseminated in the environment, learning to regulate carcinogenic chemicals may be the most urgent public health problem of the coming decades.

It is also clear that one's diet strongly influences the development of cancers. Although *how* the nature of a diet contributes to cancers of the stomach, colon, rectum, and breast is not well understood, the connection with diet is clear (Chapter 7). The hope is that research will unravel this complex problem and enable us, individually or collectively as a society, to achieve some degree of prevention through dietary practices. Research may also yield a sound basis for implementing controls over the chemical carcinogens to which we are exposed by routes other than our food and drink.

There is also evidence that one's susceptibility (or resistance) to cancer-causing agents in the environment is strongly affected by factors inherited from his or her parents (Chapter 5). Except in a few relatively rare cases, it is not known how such hereditary factors affect one's chances of developing this or that kind of cancer, although it seems likely that what we inherit is a sensitivity to one or another carcinogen or class of carcinogens. The range of such sensitivities seems to vary widely in the human population, and the study of hereditary factors may eventually enable physicians to assess *in advance* a person's susceptibilities to various carcinogens, in turn enabling the person to elect to avoid certain carcinogens and reduce his or her risk of developing cancer. That kind of capability would also form a basis for designing broad-scale programs for preventing cancer.

Identifying Carcinogens Is a Complex Task

Clearly, then, the first step toward preventing human cancer is to identify its specific causes so that they may be eliminated or avoided. Two general approaches to identification of carcinogens were discussed earlier, especially in Chapter 6: retrospective epidemiological studies and prospective laboratory tests. In epidemiological studies, human beings serve as unwitting and involuntary test animals over long periods of time and with unforeseeable consequences. The recognition that tobacco causes a variety of kinds of cancers is a prime example of the application of this methodology. Unfortunately, this particular epidemiological "experiment" continues in ever-expanding proportions even though the indictment of tobacco is unequivocal. At least some epidemiologically identified carcinogens have been eliminated or reduced: chimney soot, certain dyes, and certain industrial chemicals. In general, however, epidemiological studies are insensitive, slow, and tragically retrospective.

As a complement to epidemiological research, it is now possible to use prospective laboratory tests that involve either intact animals or cultured cells. These laboratory tests are another bounty of decades of basic research into the nature of cancer cells and their normal counterparts and offer a basis for potentially effective programs of preventing cancer.

In animal tests, the potency and actions of suspected cancer-causing agents (chemicals, radiations, and viruses) can be assessed in carefully designed experiments. The suspected agent is administered to one set of animals and the frequency of cancer in these animals is compared with the frequency in an identical set that is not exposed to the agent under study (Figure 1 in Chapter 6). Rates of administering the agents, as well as total dosage, can be varied at will. The frequencies of cancers among groups of treated and untreated animals permit a judgment about the carcinogenic effects of the agent. Such experiments are direct and can yield valuable information about the potency of a suspected carcinogen and the kinds of cancers it causes. There are, however, two inherent difficulties with this approach: one involves the difficulty of extrapolating from animals to humans and the other concerns the limited sensitivity of those animal tests.

Consider first some difficulties of extrapolating to humans information developed through animal tests of cancer-causing viruses, radiations, and chemicals. Cancer-causing viruses, for example, tend to be rather specific, affecting a narrow range of host species. Viruses that are oncogenic for rodents seem never to cause cancer in humans; viruses oncogenic for cats do not affect dogs. Studying viruses that are oncogenic for our primate relatives (apes, monkeys, lemurs) may approximate closely our own situation. Even this tactic, however, risks missing viruses that are entirely specific to humans, for example the Epstein-Barr and herpes simplex II viruses (Chapter 9).

As discussed in Chapter 8, carcinogenic radiations seem to affect the DNAs of all animals in essentially the same ways—another insight from basic research. Different species, even genetically different strains of a given species, often have somewhat different sensitivities to radiations of various kinds, but this seems to be the only significant difference among species and between humans and nonhuman animals. Thus, results from studies of the effects of radiations on animals are directly and highly relevant to the problem of radiation-induced cancers in humans.

The issue of relating results of animal tests with carcinogenic chemicals to the human situation is problematic. The problems stem from the fact that sensitivities and susceptibilities to chemical carcinogens vary greatly from species to species and from strain to strain. As mentioned in Chapter 6, rats have an enzyme that converts the precarcinogen AAF into an active carcinogen, whereas guinea pigs do not. AAF is accordingly a carcinogen for rats, but not for guinea pigs. Similarly, epidemiological studies reveal that arsenic causes cancers in humans, but repeated attempts to detect arsenic-induced cancers in test animals so far have failed (Chapter 7). Also, the poison aflatoxin is a potent carcinogen in rats and trout but apparently a less potent carcinogen in humans. Although unequivocally established, these cases tend to be exceptional: most chemical carcinogens including such common ones as benz[a]pyrene and other hydrocarbons and the various nitrosamines are carcinogenic in a broad range of species.

Animal tests must nevertheless be interpreted carefully because species do vary in their sensitivities to carcinogens, sometimes making comparisons difficult and extrapolations less than straightforward. This does not mean that the method is unsound in any serious way, although some critics of these tests would argue so. Extrapolating from animals to humans is a demonstrably useful and fruitful approach in many areas of medical research, including anesthesiology, immunology, nutrition, the physiology of mammalian organ systems, and even surgery. Much of modern medical practice derives from studies with laboratory animals, many of which are quite different from humans *except* in the features selected for study. In the context of testing for carcinogens, the issue should not be whether this or that species is a suitable animal for assessing the potency for humans of all potential carcinogens. That broad focus distorts the goal. Instead, the issue should be to determine which species are appropriate organisms for assessing a particular class of suspected carcinogens. This is the attitude medical researchers adopt in other fields, using a wide variety of animals but especially mice, rats, dogs, cats, chickens, and monkeys to study functions and diseases of particular tissues and organs. Learning which species or combination of species to use for what purpose(s) often takes decades, and modern forms of animal tests for carcinogens are only a few decades old; we are still learning. It makes no sense to reject current animal tests merely because they are not yet perfectly reliable. Whatever their momentary shortcomings, we must use them for the time being, recognizing fully that the information they yield may not be unqualifiably applicable to humans. This approach will enable researchers to accumulate the experience to evaluate the tests and thereby improve them. In time, researchers will be able to devise optimal combinations of test species and suspected agents, combinations that will provide less provisional interpretations. In the interim, simple prudence requires that substances demonstrated to be carcinogenic in current animal tests be regarded, at least potentially, as carcinogenic for humans as well.

A more fundamental shortcoming of animal tests is that they are relatively insensitive, at least under reasonable economic constraints. The issue of sensitivity concerns the number of test animals that must be used in order for the test to be truly informative. Animal tests, indeed all tests based on statistical inference, are prone to the two kinds of inherent errors shown in Table 1. The danger of falsely identifying a harmless chemical as a carcinogen, *or* of falsely identifying a carcinogen as harmless, can *never* be known in practice precisely because one cannot know in advance whether the chemical is carcinogenic or harmless: that, after all, is the purpose of the test. But by deciding in advance how large an uncertainty one is willing to accept, it is possible to determine how many animals must be used to make the test informative.

TABLE 1. Possible outcomes of tests for potential carcinogens.

Test Indicates that Agent Is:	Agent Is Actually:	
	Harmless	Carcinogenic
Harmless	Correct decision	FALSE NEGATIVE: mistakenly miss a carcinogen
Carcinogenic	FALSE POSITIVE: mistakenly indict a harmless agent	Correct decision

Assume that a given dose of some chemical increases the rate of cancer in some species from 1 to 2 percent of the animals—a fact that cannot, of course, be known in advance. To keep the risks of false positives and false negatives to 10 percent each, the test must include at least 2460 animals, half of which are exposed to the chemical. To reduce the risks of the two kinds of errors to 1 percent each would require a total of at least 6200 animals. It is possible to reduce the number of animals required to just over 4500 by accepting a 10 percent risk of a false positive, yet retaining a 1 percent risk of a false negative. Such tests would cost over $2,500,000. Notice that the social cost of a false negative—missing a true carcinogen— is potentially great. In this case an animal test that included fewer than 4500 animals but was well designed in all other respects might reasonably miss a carcinogen that increased cancer's toll by 1 percent, or by 4000 deaths annually in the United States alone.

A chemical that caused a 1 percent increase of all cancers would be classified as a significant human carcinogen. Although such carcinogens could be detected by animal tests on the scale previously described, weaker carcinogens might well escape detection. Yet identifying weak carcinogens is crucial to an effective program of preventing cancer because a substantial part of human cancer may be due to the cumulative effects of a large group of individually weak carcinogens. Suppose that a weak carcinogen that was widespread at low levels in the environment (for example, in urban air or in the food supply) was the primary cause of only 2000 out of 400,000 United States cancer deaths each year—a rate of only 5 of every 1000 cancer deaths. Such a weak carcinogen would not be detected epidemiologically and almost certainly would escape detection in animal tests of the kind so far described. One hundred such agents, each individually as weak, might in concert cause 200,000 cancer deaths—half the total.

It is thus evident that the sensitivity of animal tests for carcinogens must be maximized if the tests are to be useful for preventing cancer. There are two principal ways to achieve this. One way is to use larger numbers of animals but, as just discussed, this is too costly. The other way is to increase the effect of the chemical being tested, either by using animals that have been bred to be highly susceptible to cancer or by using large doses of the chemical.

Using test animals that are very susceptible to cancer is not as straightforward an approach as it may seem at first. The higher susceptibility might well result in a higher rate of cancers among the untreated (control) animals—cancers that are induced by extraneous or unidentified causes. This might reduce, even cancel, the advantage of using extrasusceptible animals.

Using very large doses of the chemical being tested is generally a more effective means for increasing the effectiveness of animal tests. If in the example used earlier (risk of false positives at 10 percent; risk of false negatives at 1 percent), the rate of cancer can be raised from 1 percent among the untreated controls to 10 percent among the animals treated with a very large dose, the number of animals needed for an informative test falls to just over 160, compared with 4500. For this reason, most animal tests employ the maximum dose of the test substance that does not poison or otherwise injure the treated animals, except by being carcinogenic.

In interpreting such tests, we must assume that substances that cause cancers at high doses in test animals also cause cancers at low doses in humans. This compounds the uncertainties of extrapolating from test animals to humans considered earlier. It also leaves unresolved the crucial issue of thresholds: is there, in fact, a threshold dose of each proved carcinogen below which the substance causes no human cancers? This question is extraordinarily important because many people are chronically exposed to known carcinogens at doses that fall below the levels in which routine animal tests are informative. Until it can be proved that there are safe, subthreshold levels of carcinogens, simple prudence demands that one avoid as far as possible all exposure to such substances.

It is in this context that short-term screening tests such as the Ames test (Chapter 6) become especially useful. With all their shortcomings, bacterial tests can, by measuring accurately the mutagenicity of a substance, provide an indication of its potential as a carcinogen for humans. Several other short-term tests, more or less based on the model provided by the Ames test, have been developed and are now being improved. One set of tests of potentially great value involves the detection of mutations and other kinds of genetic damage (breaking of chromosomes) in cultured animal cells, including human cells; these cultured cells can be exposed to suspected carcinogens just as the Ames test exposes bacterial cells. Such tests are also quick, relatively inexpensive, and more sensitive than animal tests, but less sensitive than bacterial tests. Although less sensitive, short-term tests with cultured animal or human cells may provide a more direct assessment of mutagenicity. It seems reasonable to anticipate for the relatively near future the development of more sensitive tests that are based on the Ames prototype but are more capable of assessing accurately the mutagenicity to humans of suspicious chemicals and other agents. Substances that are not mutagenic in such short-term tests may, at least provisionally, be regarded as no serious threat. Substances that are provisionally revealed as mutagens by short-term tests can then be analyzed in animal tests of large enough scale to determine with the necessary sensitivity whether the substance is carcinogenic. Such a two-tiered approach will not be foolproof but will optimize the use of the limited human and material resources that our society is willing and able to allocate to the search for environmental carcinogens. Indeed, such a two-tiered plan has been recommended by the National Cancer Institute.[3]

You Can Reduce Your Risk of Cancer

The message of the preceding overview of the scientific search for carcinogens is clear. Although most of the basic knowledge needed to make such a search sensitive and efficient is available, unambiguous practical techniques are not yet at hand. For each increment of speed and convenience and for each decrement of cost, there is a price. The price is a reduction of directness, that is, an increase in the psychological distance between the test organisms and living human beings. Inevitably, this generates uncertainty about how to extrapolate the test data to humans in the real world; and this, in turn, makes effective social planning difficult. Evaluating these trade-offs is only partly a matter of science. In the final analysis, the decision on how much ambiguity is acceptable is social and economic as well as scientific.

The social issue is obvious. If it is already known that a handful of environmental agents cause most human cancer, then why have these carcinogens not already been removed from the human environment? It seems far more sensible to prevent cancer than to try to cure it, particularly since present treatments are usually traumatic, sometimes life-threatening, and can cure on the average only about one victim in four. Prevention, however, is not so simple as it might first appear. Our society has not yet genuinely committed itself to preventing cancer in the way it has committed itself to preventing such infectious diseases as polio and smallpox. One commentator expressed the situation in this way:

If one thousand people died every day of cholera, swine flu, or food poisoning, an epidemic of major proportions would be at hand and the entire country would mobilize against it. Yet cancer claims that many lives daily, often in prolonged and agonizing pain, and most people believe they can do nothing about it.[4]

IMPORTANT AMBIGUITIES WILL PERSIST

If science could unequivocally identify every avoidable environmental carcinogen, the path to programs of prevention would be clear. After all, long-standing social policies prohibit (1) the introduction of poisons such as arsenic and mercury into foods; (2) bacteria that cause typhus, cholera, and other infectious diseases in both food and water; and (3) TNT and heavy weapons in general commerce. But the present state of the art does not permit such unequivocal identification of all environmental carcinogens, and the ambiguities are likely to persist, at least for some time.

The basic problem is that not all environmental agents fall into clearly definable, exclusive categories: carcinogens and noncarcinogens. Rather, research reveals a number of agents that seem questionably carcinogenic. Moreover, even in the cases of unambiguously identified carcinogens, many variables may modify the risk to particular individuals: dose rate, total dosage, duration of exposure, route of exposure, age, general health, interactions with other carcinogens and even noncarcinogenic chemicals, hereditary predisposition to cancer, and perhaps others. So to the expectable social and economic debate that surrounds the regulation of even proved carcinogens must be added an additional layer of ambiguity because science is not now and will probably never be absolutely certain of which substances are carcinogenic to every individual under every circumstance. There is no point in regretting this situation and no reason to resist setting up interim criteria for making decisions, provisional standards by which to act while waiting for the worst uncertainties to be resolved. Individuals and societies often must act without complete and final knowledge—and often do. Not to do so in the case of cancer is senseless.

Even where specific environmental sources have been identified, efforts to eliminate them from the human environment have, more often than not, been merely half-hearted. The most notorious example of this failure to prevent dissemination and use of a known, potent, and highly lethal source of carcinogens is that of tobacco. Consumption of cigarettes continues to rise, and the death rate from lung cancer continues to rise along with it (Figure 7C in Chapter 1). Many cigarette smokers are unable or unwilling to relinquish the practice. Most smokers profess a desire to give up smoking but claim that doing so is difficult. For some people, the addiction to tobacco seems to be stronger than addiction to heroin. A study commissioned by the British government has revealed, for example, that a typical youngster who had smoked more than one cigarette had only a 15 percent chance of remaining a nonsmoker.[5] Yet the addiction can be broken: 30 million Americans have stopped smoking tobacco. It is tragic that both governments and private agencies seem incapable of initiating measures adequate to reduce cigarette smoking even further. Curtailing the tobacco industry would have large, short-term, political and economic impacts. The price for refusing to accept or otherwise cope with those impacts is enormous: hundreds of thousands of premature deaths from cancer; hundreds of thousands of premature deaths from heart, lung, and circulatory diseases; and billions of dollars in needless medical costs. Yet tobacco remains unregulated and at the same time one of the most thoroughly confirmed of all carcinogens.

Preventing cancer will be costly, just as dams, sanitation, and vaccinations are costly. But those costs are accepted as part of our cultural obligations. Why cannot the costs of preventing cancer, which will be minor over the long run, also be accepted?

GOVERNMENT (IN)ACTIONS TO PREVENT CANCER

The Federal Government has already enacted a number of measures intended to protect the United States population against environmental carcinogens. The Food, Drug, and Cosmetic Act of 1938 established the regulatory authority of the Food and Drug Administration (FDA) according to which no food may be marketed that contains a "natural or added substance which may render it injurious to health." The Act has been expanded by a number of amendments, including the Delaney Amendment of 1958, according to which no substance may be added to food if it has been found to induce cancer in humans or animals. Under the Act and its amendments the FDA has banned a number of potential carcinogens including chloroform, safrole, cyclamate, and Red Dyes #2 and #4. However, the overall performance of the FDA has been less than aggressively effective in removing carcinogens from food, drugs, and cosmetics.[6]

The U.S. Department of Agriculture (USDA) has the responsibility for monitoring agricultural and meat products for pesticides and other carcinogenic contaminants. Such monitoring has contributed to a ban on DDT, dieldrin, and a number of other pesticides. But the USDA has been severely criticized for failing to monitor rigorously agricultural products, meat, and poultry for a wide variety of other pesticides and drugs and for failure to enforce high standards with respect to food contaminants, many of which are carcinogenic or otherwise injurious to health.[6] In particular, the Agency has been dilatory in regulating the exposure of United States citizens to agricultural chemicals that are banned in this country, exported to other countries, and reimported on many foods.

The Environmental Protection Agency (EPA), established in 1970, has considerable authority to control carcinogens in the environment under a variety of laws, including the Clean Air Act, the Water Pollution Control Act, the Insecticide, Fungicide, and Rodenticide Act, the Safe Drinking Water Act, and the Toxic Substances Control Act. Perhaps the most important of these is the Toxic Substances Control Act, which became law in 1976 and which was vigorously opposed by the United States chemical industry. In one major respect this law represents a turning point with regard to regulation of the hundreds of thousands of chemicals now produced and spread into the human environment. The law shifts the burden of proof from the general public to the manufacturers and disseminators of chemicals. In effect, it requires a manufacturer to prove that a given chemical is safe rather than requiring the public, through the government or another organization, to prove that it is harmful.

Another important development was the implementation in 1980 of the Resource Conservation and Recovery Act. This legislation requires careful accounting of all toxic and hazardous materials, from the point of manufacture to ultimate disposal. The intention is to inhibit or prevent unsafe methods of handling and disposing of potentially dangerous materials.

The Occupational Safety and Health Administration (OSHA) was created by Congress in 1970 to be part of the Department of Labor and was charged with assuring as far as possible safe and healthful working conditions for all American workers. OSHA has set standards to minimize exposure of workers to several carcinogens, notably asbestos (1972), vinyl chloride (1974), coke-oven emissions (1976), and benzene (1978).[6] However, as one can see from the list of occupationally related cancers in Table 4 in Chapter 7, a considerable task remains to remove carcinogens from the American workplace.

Overall, then, a number of steps have been taken by the

Federal Government to remove or limit some carcinogens in the environment. However, the action of governmental agencies under the various laws has been slow and limited compared to what might be done on the basis of current knowledge. In large measure this slow progress is the result of enormous pressures exerted on Congress and governmental agencies by special interest groups that might, in the short run, be adversely affected by vigorous programs to prevent cancer. In the glaring case of prevention of tobacco carcinogenesis, the minimal action of the Federal Government toward prevention has been more than negated by its counterproductive support of the tobacco industry.

Another aspect of the Government's relative ineffectiveness may stem from reluctance to act when the case against one or another environmental carcinogen is not unequivocally proved. The reluctance in the case of cancer is not new, having surfaced in the past with other regulatory issues now generally accepted, such as chlorination and fluoridation of drinking water, and vaccination. This reluctance is often compounded by debates over the evidence for or against the carcinogenicity of individual substances and practices. A more constructive approach would be to establish general criteria and rules of evidence for assessing carcinogenicity, recognizing that such guidelines initially would be provisional. Only then can a consistent policy for preventing preventable cancer be put in place. And it must be remembered that not to decide on such guidelines is to decide to tolerate preventable cancers.

In summary, the efforts of the Federal Government in preventing cancer are piecemeal, uncoordinated, and almost always vigorously opposed for economic reasons by one or another manufacturing, agricultural, or other industry or its organizational representatives. The tragedy of this situation can be measured by the hundreds of thousands of people who will suffer and die of cancer caused by already identified environmental carcinogens that could be controlled or eliminated. Given these realities, prudent personal actions and behaviors are an individual's first line of defense against cancer.

PERSONAL ACTIONS CAN BE EFFECTIVE

In the absence of an effective and uncompromising governmental program to reduce or eliminate carcinogens from the human environment, we can as individuals do much to minimize our own exposures to carcinogens. Most environmental carcinogens so far identified have proved to be chemicals, although ultraviolet radiation in sunlight, medical X rays, and radioactive materials all account for a significant number of largely preventable cancers. Each year, new chemicals are added to the list of suspected or proved carcinogens. The list has now grown so long and is so varied (see Chapter 7) as to elicit from some persons reactions of despair, sometimes epitomized by the statement, "We live in a sea of carcinogens." Even by pessimistic standards, this is an exaggeration. One may never be able to avoid all carcinogens all of the time, but by following a few prudent rules, one can easily avoid needless exposure to most known carcinogens, particularly the most potent ones, most of the time. Because the risk of developing cancer is probably determined by the total accumulated exposure to all carcinogens over a lifetime, each avoidance helps to reduce the personal risk of cancer.

It is also emphatically not true that "enough of anything will cause cancer." Nearly all established carcinogens act in biochemically definite ways on DNA or on other cellular constituents. There is no need to destroy our technological agriculture or our industrialized society in the quest to avoid cancer. In the few cases where acceptable substitutes for demonstrated carcinogens are not immediately at hand, we can rely on the ingenuity of the chemical industry and the efficient operation of market forces to provide innocuous, or at least safer, equivalents.

The most important and most often overlooked fact is that most carcinogens to which humans are exposed do not occur naturally in the human environment or at least are not an inevitable part of the environment. Most carcinogens have been added by some form of human activity or enterprise. These include chemical contaminants in food, water, and air; occupational exposure to chemicals, for example, asbestos, aniline dyes, certain metals, wood dust, and various other industrial fumes and chemicals; and radioactive dusts in uranium mines. Some cancers result from medical exposure to X rays. The imprudent use of X rays that in the past caused much needless cancer among radiologists and their patients continues, although on a much smaller scale. Unjustified exposure to X rays (for example, in treating nonthreatening diseases or conditions, such as ringworm, and acne) remains an important problem. The diagnostic or therapeutic value of routine X rays is still often far outweighed by the cancer risk incurred by their use, but every use of X rays must be scrutinized for its benefit/risk ratio.

There are, of course, some carcinogenic agents in the environment that are not introduced by human activity. For example, most skin cancer is caused by excessive exposure to sunlight over many years; however, the prevention of such cancers is, in principle, simple. Carcinogenic chemicals are normal constituents of certain foods, and these are perhaps less easily avoided. But in sum, most, probably nearly all cancer results from exposure to identifiable carcinogens that could be eliminated from the environment or could be avoided to a significant degree. The state of present knowledge as presented in this book provides a basis for personal actions that can effectively reduce the personal risk of cancer. Don't smoke; drink alcohol only in moderation (and never when you smoke, if you must); avoid nonessential X rays and other forms of radiation, including excessive sunlight; eat a low-fat, high-fiber diet; avoid carcinogenic foods, such as charred foods and charred meat in particular; avoid occupations that entail exposure to known carcinogens (Tables 1 through 5 in Chapter 7). These few, relatively simple adjustments in life-style will substantially reduce the likelihood that you will develop an avoidable cancer.

There is no way to remove every last carcinogen from our communal environment. Even if this became a social goal, cancer could not thereby be completely eliminated. Cosmic rays, sunlight, background radiation, and thermal noise in replicating DNA will always cause some irreducible minimum of cancer. But a society can choose to control most carcinogens and prevent most cancer, reducing drastically the current rate of 1100 deaths per day in the United States alone. Preventing cancer will require a combination of scientific achievement, social courage, and prudent personal behaviors. The key to the problem is an informed public that can exercise its influence.

Remain informed by reading beyond this book and use the information you acquire to protect yourself in other ways. Interpret skeptically reports from all sources of the danger or safety of this or that material or practice. Be especially skeptical of reports that do not stipulate that the test described was statistically powerful enough to be informative. Statistics alone cannot reveal the truth of any situation, but statistics can place possible errors and uncertainties into perspective. Be skeptical, for example, of reports that no excess cancers were observed among the treated animals: the absence of evidence is not evidence of absence.

Above all, express yourself as a citizen and as a consumer. Social changes of the kind necessary to prevent avoidable cancer will soon follow if enough people vote in the marketplace as well as at the ballot box.

Psychosocial Aspects of Cancer

Laurie Engelberg & Lee Hilborne

EVEN if an enlightened and effective program of preventing cancer were put into effect immediately, cancer would continue to strike many people for some decades to come. People exposed to carcinogens today may not develop clinically detectable disease for many years, and eliminating all major known carcinogens will still leave minor known carcinogens as well as those not yet recognized.

Cancer will thus remain a problem for the foreseeable future and will have to be reckoned with, coped with. Chapter 10 outlined the main current medical treatments available to cancer patients, and Chapter 11 explored some of the social and political aspects of the cancer problem. Here are emphasized the psychological and personal impact of the disease on the patient and his or her family, friends, and co-workers.

Delaying Treatment Is Common and Dangerous

Delay can be fatal when dealing with cancer. As explained in Chapter 10, the earlier a cancer is detected, the less likely it is that metastasis has occurred, and the more likely it is that treatment may contain the disease.[1] Not all cancers can be detected early, but for those that can be, survival rates are improved when the patient seeks medical help promptly. Breast cancer in women can in many instances be detected through a simple and convenient monthly self-examination.[2] Among women whose breast cancers were detected early and treated while still localized, the 5-year survival rate was 85 percent. By contrast, the 5-year survival rate was only 56 percent among women whose breast cancers had spread.[3] Cancers of the colon and rectum may be signaled by rectal bleeding, and rectal cancers are often discovered by the physician's touch. Five-year survival rates for these cancers drop from over 70 percent when treated while still localized to only 40 percent in men and 47 percent in women when the cancer has become regional.[3] These and other cancers may be signaled by the widely advertised CAUTION signs listed in Chapter 10; but even when people recognize the possible significance of one of these signs, many will delay seeking medical help.

Such delay behavior is hardly unique to cancer, but the delays seem to be longer for symptoms associated with cancer than for symptoms associated with other diseases.[4] This tendency to delay longer in the face of suspected cancer probably reflects a variety of fears about the disease, some justified, others not. Many cancer patients worry about the ways family, friends, and co-workers might react to them after receiving news of a cancer. Others dread the unpredictability of the disease or the disfigurement that may result either directly from the disease or indirectly from amputation or chemotherapy. And of course, the overriding fear of death is commonplace. Other emotions reported by persons who postponed seeking medical evaluation of suspected symptoms of cancer include guilt over past negligence and over having delayed seeking help; shame and modesty over the site of the suspected cancer; and pessimism and fatalism.[5,6]

Another factor that contributes to delay in obtaining help is ignorance of symptoms that may point to cancer. Even individuals who appreciate the relation of certain symptoms to cancer may procrastinate because they underestimate the potential seriousness of the symptoms. Denial, either of the possible significance of symptoms or of the possible seriousness of the disease, also accounts for delaying behaviors.[4,7] In general, persons who are more aware of cancer-related symptoms tend to procrastinate less than those who are not.[8] Understandably, persons who have experienced cancer among family or friends often procrastinate longer than those who have not.[6,9]

An individual's attitudes toward and relationships with physicians can also affect his or her reactions. Weak or poor doctor-patient relationships are associated with prolonged delays in seeking medical help, whereas strongly positive relationships generally influence rapid, effective responses to suspected symptoms of cancer.[6]

Studies of reactions to suspicions of cancer reveal that several social and demographic attributes are commonly associated with delaying behaviors. On the average, persons who are older, less wealthy, and with less formal education tend to delay action longer than do younger, affluent persons with more formal education. Education may be the essential factor here, underlying correlations between delay and other characteristics studied.[6] Delays in obtaining medical help may also reflect the way the health care system is organized and operated.[10] Health care facilities are often staffed by relatively young members of the middle class who may find it easier to provide medical treatment for persons like themselves. Health care systems are also organized to serve most efficiently those who will use them, and the middle class and affluent segments of our society make more use of the system than do their less affluent counterparts. Finally, patients need certain social skills to use the system effectively—assertiveness, persistence, self-confidence—and older, less educated persons may not have these skills or even realize that they are needed. Accordingly, they may be less able to make the system work for them and less inclined to try.

Whatever the reasons, many people do not act promptly when faced with evidence of possible cancer. Such behavior is unwise and dangerous, usually leading to a less favorable prognosis when medical help is eventually sought. The message is clear: people must be educated about the importance of detecting cancer early, and also need to be convinced of the importance of acting promptly when suspicious signs arise. More immediately, we must each have the courage to seek medical help promptly and must urge those close to us to do the same.

Reactions to the Diagnosis Vary

The diagnosis of a cancer can be a devastating emotional blow to the patient and to the patient's family and friends. Because the diagnosis itself may disrupt the lives of many, cancer practitioners—physicians, nurses, social workers, technicians—are concerned over how to convey a diagnosis of cancer. Before the 1960s, physicians seldom told their patients that they had cancer. For example, one study conducted in 1960 revealed that only 12 percent of the medical staff of a Chicago hospital consistently informed their patients of diagnoses of cancer and that even they conveyed diagnoses through euphemisms such as "growth," "hyperplastic tissue," and "lesion."[11] This was so even though a study published a decade earlier showed that more than 80 percent of 200 patients asserted that they would want to be informed if they were diagnosed as having cancer.[12]

More recently, it has become common practice to inform most patients of the nature of their illness.[13] The manner in which the diagnosis of cancer is communicated is crucial because the disease is often equated not only with death but with a kind of living and dying that involves chronic disability, dependence, and pain. The task of informing patients of the diagnosis usually falls to the physician. It is a difficult task, one not always accomplished with distinction. Many patients view the reporting physician not merely as a reporter of unwelcome medical facts but as a sentence-giver, an executioner.[6] Recognizing this, the physician must decide carefully how much to disclose, in what manner, and how soon. A sensitive physician will try to respond to cues from the patient about appropriate levels of explanation, especially about the effects of unfamiliar or potentially threatening terms, and will try to assess the patient's capacity to absorb information. A physician may elect to devote more than a single session to explaining the diagnosis, proposed treatments, and prognosis. Attempting to balance honesty with sensitivity, the physician will try to help sustain hope while remaining truthful, equally avoiding undue pessimism or optimism. Because patients may fail to understand the significance of diagnoses that are optimistically or gently conveyed, even sensitive physicians may need to resort to frank, even strong, language.

Unfortunately, even when a physician attempts to balance these conflicting demands, behavior may not match intentions. A major constraint is that medical training encourages a degree of detachment in the physician, a detachment that may indeed be essential for the physician's emotional survival. Consequently, physicians are often not prepared, either by nature or by training, to respond sensitively to terminally ill patients, be they victims of cancer or another ailment.[13] Nor are physicians immune to the deadly images evoked by the word cancer, and they may feel virtually helpless when confronted with certain forms of the disease.[14] Such feelings may well impair the physician's psychological capacity to deal sensitively with some patients. Nevertheless, most patients want to be informed not only of their diagnosis, but also of the details of all proposed treatments.[12,13]

Patient and physician are not the only parties who must come to grips with the diagnosis of cancer. The patient's cancer and required treatments inevitably impinge on the lives of those closest to the patient. Unable to address their own feelings of inadequacy, frustrated relatives may criticize the patient, blaming him or her for prior behavior that presumably caused the cancer.[13] Such reactions from loved ones can clearly devastate the patient. Conversely, family and friends have opportunities to play positive and productive roles in the patient's future. Open and honest communication among the patient and those close to him or her is usually valuable for all.[15] Indeed, stability and cohesiveness within the family can be enhanced by sharing the diagnosis, even to the point of having patient and family together when it is disclosed.[13] This ensures that nothing about the diagnosis is secret or withheld. This kind of supportive openness can lay the basis for coping with the cancer as a family, not just an individual, problem. Sadly, these opportunities are not always realized. In general, family relationships following a diagnosis of cancer are quite similar to those that existed before the diagnosis; strong loving families are often able to cope with stresses imposed by catastrophic illnesses, whereas such stresses invariably make matters worse in families that are already weak and strained.[15]

Regardless of how much the fact of the cancer affects others in the family, the cancer patient is obviously the person most affected by the diagnosis and by the disease. A patient's reactions to a diagnosis of cancer depend on many things, including how the diagnosis is revealed. Generally, the patient's reactions depend upon the strength of her or his ego and personality and are inevitably similar to the person's reactions during previous life-threatening crises.[15]

The initial response to the confirmation of cancer is often emotional turmoil. This reaction may be expressed as disbelief, anger, or depression and may be accompanied by grief, anxiety, insomnia, loss of appetite, an inability to concentrate, and irritability.[16] Fears aroused in the patient may include those associated with death, uncertainty over the future, fear of pain, fear of losing body parts or bodily functions, worries over impending loss of family and work roles, fear of dependency, concern over the cost of treatment, and fear of alienation from others.[16] At this initial stage, most cancer victims need to express these kinds of emotions, to verbalize what they are feeling about their disease and the life that remains. Well-meaning friends and relatives sometimes talk more and offer more advice than is useful at this stage, behaviors that may inadvertently further confuse and isolate the patient. Instead, family members (and health professionals) should listen, encouraging the patient to express her or his feelings, and being alert for the cues and hints the patient offers about emotional wants and needs. Such appropriate behaviors often ease tensions on all sides, enabling all to cope more openly and directly with the disease and its impacts.

One final issue needs to be considered in connection with the diagnosis phase of cancer. Once the diagnosis has been made, treatment is likely to begin as soon as feasible; given the nature of the disease, immediate treatment is invariably a good idea. However, physicians are not infallible, and because the side effects of treating cancer can be serious, the patient has a right to seek a second opinion on both the diagnosis and the proposed course of treatment—even if this delays temporarily the start of treatment. It is important for individuals to take full advantage of the health care system in this way and not to let doctors, or the system itself, coerce or intimidate them into precipitate action, especially if that action (e.g., an amputation) is to be irreversible.

Cancer's Consequences Are Also Varied

The clinical course of the disease exposes the cancer patient to a variety of physical and emotional assaults that call for major psychological adjustments. Among the major stresses that challenge the patient's capacity to cope are the effects of the cancer itself on the body; the effects of the treatments; the structure of the medical care system; and the responses by others to the cancer patient.

Many cancer patients are clinically depressed, yet it is unclear to what extent depression is a result of the disease itself and to what extent it is a function of the consequences of the disease: treatments, loss of jobs, ostracism, and other social changes.[17] Depression is more evident among older cancer patients, whereas anger is the emotional response most often expressed by the young. Other emotional reactions to cancer include exaggeration of personality traits, exaggeration of physical symptoms, guilt, anxiety, insomnia, tendencies to retreat from problems, and possibly even psychotic behavior.[6,15,18,19] These are all understandable responses in light of the life-threatening nature of the illness.

Pain is less common among cancer patients than is depression; only about one-third of all cancer victims suffer significant pain.[20] Nevertheless, pain is a very important aspect of cancer, particularly for patients suffering from untreatable cancers.

Pain must also be controlled with large doses of narcotics, drugs some health professionals are reluctant to use because they are addicting. But for terminally ill patients, drug addiction cannot be an issue. Pain can thus be controlled by providing adequate amounts of narcotics and other medications at regular intervals. The aim here is to prevent disease-related pain rather than removing pain as it develops. This is especially important in that both the patient's mood and behavior are eroded by recurrent pain. If pain can be averted, the quality of the patient's remaining life will be enhanced, a reasonable and humane goal. Strategies for controlling pain in patients not considered terminally ill are more controversial. Most physicians will attempt to offer the maximum relief consistent with avoiding addiction to pain-killing narcotics. Many physicians will also risk transient addiction because without effective medication, their patients' pain might become virtually intolerable.

Treatments for cancer can be so formidable that they are sometimes thought to be worse than the disease: surgery may involve the loss of a body part or function; radiation and chemotherapy are known to cause the temporary loss of hair, severe nausea, and diarrhea. Such highly stressful treatments are sometimes better tolerated by the optimistic patient who believes that a cure can be achieved.[16,21]

Treatments for cancer often require hospitalization, which exposes the patient to an additional set of psychological stresses. A hospital environment allows a retreat from the responsibilities and problems of life, and the structure of the institution tends to force the patient into nearly total dependence. The hospitalized cancer patient, like all hospitalized patients, must frequently rely on the benevolence of hospital personnel, physician, and family for even the most basic care, an often difficult and demeaning situation. Another psychological stress on hospitalized patients stems from being isolated from friends and family during the hospitalization.

When hospitalization ends, cancer may bring about changes in the patient's social roles, changes that require profound and stressful adjustments. Friends and acquaintances are liable to treat the patient differently, to interact in strained and uncomfortable ways. Friends and co-workers who, with good intentions, treat cancer patients as if they are fragile or delicate may unintentionally imply that the patient can never again be normal or productive. In addition, well-meaning curiosity about any illness may be unwelcome, especially for cancer patients attempting to resume normal life styles.

Cancer's aftermath can be disorienting for the entire family. Being hospitalized for an extended period or being temporarily or permanently disabled after leaving the hospital may prevent the cancer patient from resuming his or her former position in the family, from meeting the family's traditional expectations as mother, father, or other relative. Because the family must continue to function, roles and tasks previously the responsibility of the cancer patient are necessarily taken over by others, often while the patient is still being cared for, either in the hospital or at home. These adjustments may inadvertently redefine the role of the patient in ways that evoke guilt and feelings of inadequacy, even worthlessness.[18]

Some cancer patients suffer permanent physical disfigurements that impose new social roles, some highly stressful. Head and neck cancers can be particularly debilitating in a society like ours in which physical attractiveness is so valued. For example, cancer of the larynx (voicebox) may require removal of the larynx (laryngectomy) so that normal speech becomes impossible. Subsequently, the patient can speak only by swallowing air and forcing it back up through the throat and air passages behind the nose in a kind of controlled burp. A low-pitched sound, the patient's new voice, is produced as the air in these passages vibrates. Artificial electronic voiceboxes are also available.[22] Surgical removal of certain forms of cancer frequently impairs or destroys sexual functions, for example, cancers of the testes or prostate in men and some cancers of the vagina, cervix, or uterus in women. Even when sexual functions are not physiologically impaired, the psychological ramifications of cancer may prevent normal erotic relationships. For example, one quarter of women who have undergone a mastectomy (removal of a breast) report subsequent sexual disturbances, as do about half of the men who have undergone colostomies (creation of an opening from the colon through the body wall through which wastes can be voided).[23] In either case, these sexual dysfunctions may impose intense emotional stresses on patients and on their sexual partners.

Social stresses also assault the cancer patient from outside the family circle. Given the aura of mystery with which many people still regard cancer, it isn't surprising that myths abound in the lay population. Although no evidence supports fear that human cancers are contagious, this misconception is firmly entrenched. Consequently, patients are often ostracized, even long after a cancer has been controlled or gone into remission.

Another context for cancer-connected social stress involves employment. Employers are often reluctant to hire cancer patients, claiming, for example, that they cannot afford the cost of training workers who may not be able to remain on the job very long. Because of this, many employers formerly invoked a "5-year rule," which stipulated that cancer patients could not be hired unless their cancers had been in remission for at least that long. Work is more than an economic necessity for most people, it is a way of life, a source of self-esteem, and an important source of social status. For the cancer patient, returning to work may symbolize returning to a normal life-style.[7] Records of performance and absenteeism among cancer patients who have returned to work compare favorably with those of other employees. Refusing to employ people who have had cancer is thus a waste of human resources. These facts are recognized in the Federal Rehabilitation Act of 1973, which protects the vocational rights of cancer patients.[24]

Some cancer patients are not concerned about discrimination in the workplace because the aftermath of their disease makes it impossible for them to return to work. In addition to the psychological stress this imposes, this presents a problem of lost income, one of the many financial burdens encountered by cancer patients and their families. Other expenses associated with cancer include medical bills, transportation costs during outpatient periods, the costs of living away from home if such a move is necessary to obtain treatment, and, perhaps, funeral and burial expenses. For patients with advanced cancers, during the early 1970s these costs ranged up to $50,000 over the course of the disease, but tended to be nearer $22,000 on the average.[25]

This section has touched on many psychological and social stresses that affect cancer patients and those close to them. Many other consequences could be added if space allowed: persistent fears of recurrences of the disease; difficulties of adjusting to prosthetic devices and other restrictions; emotional consequences of divorces precipitated by disease-related stresses; and, in familes in which the cancer patient is a child, problems caused by neglecting other children. These are relatively common consequences.

Two relatively uncommon responses to cancer deserve mention here, even if only briefly. The first is the recourse to unproven and unorthodox methods of cancer therapy, most notably the material known as laetrile. Orthodox treatments for cancer do involve distressing side effects and are not spectacularly successful overall; and for a distressing number of cancer patients, medical science stands helpless. Unproven methods may well seem mild and attractive by comparison. It should not be surprising that each year tens of thousands of patients with cancer turn to treatments that promise not to "burn, poison, or mutilate." The problem is that unproven methods are just that, unproven. Should the unproven method fail, as they generally do, patients may return to conventional treatments at a stage of their disease when conventional treatment is even less effective than it might have been earlier. The tragedy consists of time and opportunity lost.

The second uncommon response to cancer, one which may amount to a strategy for coping with the disease, is suicide. Although only a small minority of all cancer victims choose to terminate their lives, the suicide rate among cancer patients is considerably higher than among the general population. For example, 25 percent of all persons who commit suicide in hospitals are cancer patients, who make up only 12 percent of the hospitalized population.[26] Persons facing uncertainty or facing the certainty of a painful death may regard suicide as a wholly comprehensible option. These realities highlight the need for adequate systems of psychological support, the means to help cancer patients during the final phases of their afflictions, a topic considered later in this chapter.

Death and Dying Can Be Eased and Dignified

Because only one third or fewer of all patients with newly diagnosed malignant tumors can be cured, no overview of the psychological aspects of cancer can avoid issues related to death and dying.

Once a patient's disease is considered to be incurable (i.e., terminal), that person's self-image and relationships with others are radically altered, sometimes leading to what social scientists call "symbolic death" of the patient, a complex set of emotional and social changes that may precede biological death by many weeks.[27] Most patients confronted with their own impending mortality express a sense of powerlessness, loss of control, an often greater apprehension over the process of dying than over death itself.[28] Patients with terminal cancer may engage in or be placed in what social scientists call the "dying role," which imposes expectations beyond those imposed by the "sick role." Patients in the sick role are temporarily released from ordinary social responsibilities, are expected to seek competent medical help, and to cooperate in the process of trying to become well again (although getting well is not seen as an act of will alone). Patients in the dying role are also released from ordinary responsibilities and are also expected to accept all competent medical support, including losses of privacy and freedom those may entail. Further, the dying role recognizes that there will be no recovery, either from the disease or from the role. It also imposes additional expectations on the patient: to want to remain alive; to remain as independent as possible for as long as the disease permits; and to accept responsibility for permanently transferring social roles and obligations to others ("getting one's affairs in order").[29]

Patients with incurable diseases, including cancer, may have special needs, needs that although universal are intensified by their immediate circumstances. Perhaps their most important need, one already alluded to, is for the control of their pain, which may become chronic and excruciating. Surgery and medication are the most common medical interventions for controlling pain, and each carries some disadvantages and risks. Palliative surgery is often effective, for example, colostomies for patients with obstructed bowels, or severing the nerves to affected organs or tissues. Unfortunately, such interventions often extend a patient's hospitalization at the very stage of their illness at which terminally ill patients could best participate in their community. Drugs, particularly narcotic analgesics such as cocaine and morphine, cause altered states of consciousness, again impairing final exchanges between patients and those for whom they care.

A second important need of patients with advanced cancer is that for dignity. Feelings of dignity stem from a person's sense of control over self and environment and are at least as important following a diagnosis of incurable disease as at any other stage of life. So are feelings of privacy and autonomy: also basic human needs that are intensified in cases of terminal illness. But people in the process of dying are often forced to spend considerable time in hospitals—institutions designed to diagnose and treat acute disease, institutions set up to serve the sick rather than the dying. Hospitals are institutionally unable to provide the very kind of flexible and tolerant care dying patients and those close to them have a right to expect. This is not to condemn hospitals but only to point out the essential mismatch between what is needed and what is available to a special group of patients. As described in the following section, this mismatch is being addressed by new kinds of institutions, the hospices.

Many dying patients express fears of loneliness and of separation from loved ones and friends, revealing a third need, that for love and affection. The patient needs to be reassured, in word and deed, that he or she will not be abandoned or forsaken by the healthy. Maintaining physical contact is one important way to provide this reassurance, but love is also listening, perceiving, and following the patient's cues.[30] When communications of this kind taper off, depression, loneliness, and despair invariably ensue.[31]

Society in general and the medical community in particular

have long acted on the belief that human life, in any form, must be preserved whenever possible. To this end, numerous devices and high-level technologies are used to sustain and artificially extend the lives of patients: mechanical ventilators (respirators), cardiac pressure monitors, dialysis machines, and others. This attitude glosses over the more fundamental issue of the *quality* of the life being sustained. The crucial and unresolved question is whether artificial intervention in the care of the dying prolongs life or prolongs only the act of dying.[32]

Public pressure to curb the artificial maintenance of life beyond some reasonable expectation for recovery has prompted procedures under which a patient may elect, prior to the appointed time, to have life-extending treatments withheld. The "Living Will" of the Living Will Society of New York, which specifically requests that no heroics be used in case of a terminal illness, is not a legally binding document. California's Natural Death Act of 1976 provides for Directives to Physicians that enable patients to instruct health professionals to withhold heroic measures, to permit an imminent death to proceed naturally. These Directives can be legally binding on California's physicians when certain conditions are met. Similar legislation is in effect in Arkansas, Idaho, Kansas, Nevada, New Mexico, North Carolina, Oregon, Texas, and Washington, and has been introduced in other states. In growing numbers, both physicians and laypersons are electing to emphasize the quality of dying over the quantity of living.

The Hospice Movement Offers an Alternative

The concept of a humane and dignified passage into death is the philosophical foundation of Hospice. On a practical level, Hospice provides palliative care to patients suffering from terminal illnesses. Although Hospice programs do not intend to serve cancer victims alone, such patients are likely to be a majority in any given program. Hospice is a reaction against unremitting medical technology and is an effort to attend to the basic physical, emotional, and spiritual needs of dying human beings and their families.

The Hospice concept has evolved from way-stations for medieval pilgrims to modern care centers for the terminally ill. Hospices as we know them today are a result of conversations, which took place during 1948, between a dying patient and a medical social worker. The patient was acutely aware of his needs as a dying person and had visions of the kind of place that could truly have helped him in his last days. The medical social worker was Cicely Saunders. In 1967, she opened St. Christopher's Hospice, an independent health care facility in London, England.

In the Hospice philosophy, the unit of care and concern is the entire family. Family members are encouraged to participate in the care and support of the dying loved ones. They are, for example, encouraged to perform such practical services as cooking a favorite dish for the patient, administering oral medications, or helping the patient with personal hygiene. Incorporating the family into the care of the dying patient is as important for the family as for the patient. By spending time with the patient, by participating in the daily routine, the family come to feel that they have contributed to the loved one's peaceful death. This kind of participation seems to minimize guilt among survivors during their bereavement period.[30] Further, the family treatment program allows individuals the opportunity to work through their relationships with the patient before the patient's death.

In contrast to the institutionalized sterility of conventional hospitals for the acutely ill, the Hospice setting is intended to be home-like, supportive, and nurturant. Friends are encouraged to visit patients without arbitrary restrictions. Hospices use interdisciplinary teams that include physicians, nurses, clergy, lay counselors, social workers, health aides, and volunteers, all working with the entire family in a loving and caring atmosphere. These persons remain available to aid surviving relatives and friends after the patient has died.

Control of the patient's pain is perhaps the single most important goal of Hospice. According to Cicely Saunders, there is no such thing as "too much" analgesic.[30] To control the pain of dying patients, an antipain medication may be served every

4 hours around the clock. Known as Brompton's Cocktail, or Hospice Mix, it is a liquid blend of morphine, cocaine, sugar syrup, an antinausea agent, and gin. The Hospice staff attempts to provide enough analgesic to control pain without altering the patient's awareness or mental state. The required doses often decrease, once a patient's anxieties about pain are relieved.[30]

Although the prototype modern Hospice, St. Christopher's of London, is an independent unit, only some Hospices in the United States exist in this form. And although Hospice's concepts are utilized in all, much of what is termed Hospice in the United States is actually programs of extensive home care for the patient. Even in instances where Hospice does denote a particular place or institution, there is a trend away from isolated units and toward Hospice-oriented units connected with conventional medical facilities.

The Hospice movement in the United States is still young, although it grows stronger and larger daily. The long-range success of Hospice in the United States will depend on fiscal considerations as well as on how well its stated goals are met. Currently, Hospice care is less costly than roughly equivalent hospital care and in some regions is covered, at least in part, by conventional health insurance plans. There is a danger, however, that Hospices across the nation may become merely glorified nursing homes. That would be unfortunate; the Hospice concept is a socially important one because it serves a vulnerable population whose needs have in the past been largely ignored by conventional medical systems.

Support Services Are Available to All Cancer Families

Although many end-stage cancer patients can best be served through inpatient Hospice settings, most cancer patients can be aided through a network of outpatient and community services while they continue to function as members of their communities and families. To meet the escalating demand for such services, an increasing number of public and private organizations have been established.

The National Cancer Institute (NCI) in Washington, D.C., was established in 1937 as a major branch of the National Institutes of Health. A major function of the NCI is to fund community outreach programs directed at educating the public in methods of preventing, detecting, and treating cancers. As part of its mission, NCI maintains a national Cancer Information Service, which is available to all without charge. By dialing a toll-free number, the caller is put in touch with NCI personnel who will answer questions about many aspects of the diagnosis and treatment of cancer. The staff of this "Hotline" will, at the caller's request, mail to the caller helpful booklets and reference materials written for laypersons. The toll-free number for the national Cancer Hotline is 1-800-638-6694; it operates from 8 A.M. to midnight (Eastern Time) every day of the year. Certain large cities maintain local Cancer Centers, which provide similar services to the immediate community; these are listed in the appendix. Although these hotlines provide important information, they cannot replace routine physical examinations in the early detection of malignancies, nor can they replace the attending physician as a source of immediately relevant detail.

In several communities, the NCI also funds psychosocial hotlines staffed primarily by clinical psychologists specifically trained to meet the needs of persons coping with the stresses of cancer. Support is also available through local health departments, which should be contacted directly.

The forerunner of private organizations serving cancer families is the American Cancer Society (ACS), which funds basic and applied research on cancer, public education, and professional education of health care personnel. The ACS supports a network of professional and lay workers dedicated to finding effective treatments for cancer and to providing cancer patients and their families with needed support. A great deal of this energy comes from cancer patients themselves. These special volunteers provide both a special understanding and inspiration for more recently diagnosed patients who may be experiencing emotional turmoil.

One of the largest volunteer groups supported by the ACS

is Reach to Recovery, an organization of women who have had mastectomies to remove breast cancers. These volunteers visit other mastectomy patients, either in the hospital or at home during their convalescence. In addition to providing psychological support, the volunteers offer information on where prostheses are available locally and provide information and equipment for exercises essential to a complete recovery. Similar ACS-supported organizations assist victims of other kinds of cancers. Information about what ACS services are available in a particular community can be obtained by calling the Public Education or Patient Service department of a local American Cancer Society Unit (see Appendix). Other private organizations include the Ostomy Society and the Lost Chord Club. Special mention should be made of the Ronald McDonald Houses located near major cancer centers, which provide lodging so that parents may be near their children who are receiving treatment for cancer.

The foregoing outline of psychological and emotional stresses is not to be taken as a prediction or guarantee of the experiences of every patient with cancer. Rather it is an account of what can but need not happen to patients and their families, experiences that are less likely to happen if the patient and family seek the help and support of others who have already been through similar experiences or who have special training to help families struck by catastrophic diseases.

Cancer is a tragedy that taxes even the strongest egos, faiths, and relationships. As with the purely scientific aspects of cancer presented in the first 11 chapters of this book, foreknowledge of its psychological aspects is a form of power, power that may help new victims and their loved ones to cope with the emotional traumas that often follow the disease.

Notes

Chapter 1

1. Davidson, W. R. 1967. The Egyptian medical papyri. In D. Brothwell and A. T. Sandison (eds.). *Disease in Antiquity.* C. C. Thomas, Springfield, Illinois.
2. Orteaga, O. and G. T. Pack. 1966. On the antiquity of melanoma. *Cancer 19*:607–610. (This photograph is reproduced from a print kindly provided by Dr. M. B. Shimkin, University of California at San Diego School of Medicine.)
3. U.S. House of Representatives, 33rd Congress, Second Session. 1855. *Mortality Statistics of the 7th Census of the United States, 1850.* Executive Document No. 98. Washington, D.C.
4. U.S. Department of Commerce. 1976. *Historical Statistics of the United States: Colonial Times to 1970.* Washington, D.C. See also U.S. Department of Commerce. 1974–1976. *Statistical Abstracts of the United States, 1974* through *1979.* Washington, D.C.
5. U.S. Department of Health and Human Services, 1980. *Vital Statistics of the United States, 1977.* Vol. IIB. Hyattsville, Maryland.
6. From Westoff, C. F. 1974. The populations of the developed countries. *Scientific American 231*:108–120.
7. U.S. Bureau of the Census, 1978. *Current Population Reports,* Series P-25, No. 721, "Estimates of the population of the United States, by age, sex, and race: 1970–1977." U.S. Government Printing Office, Washington. See also Note 5.
8. Harris, R. H., T. Page and N. A. Reiches. 1977. Carcinogenic hazards of organic chemicals in drinking water. In H. H. Hiatt, J. D. Watson and J. A. Winsten (eds.). *Origins of Human Cancer,* Cold Spring Harbor Lab., Cold Spring Harbor, New York*, pp. 309–330.
9. Siverberg, E. and A. I. Holleb. 1973. Cancer statistics, 1973. *Ca—A Cancer Journal for Clinicians 23*:2–27.
10. The annual January/February issues of *Ca—A Cancer Journal for Clinicians* include up-to-date cancer-related statistics and trends. Refer to the issues from 1977 to date.
11. Chiazze, L. Jr., D. L. Levin and D. T. Silverman. 1977. Recent changes in estimated cancer mortality. In *Origins of Human Cancer,* pp. 33–44.

*In subsequent citations, this important collection will be referred to as *Origins of Human Cancer.*

12. Silverberg, E. 1981. Cancer statistics, 1981. *Ca—A Cancer Journal for Clinicians 31*:13–28.
13. Pollack, E. S. and J. W. Horm. 1980. Trends in cancer incidence and mortality in the United States, 1969–1976. *J. Natl. Cancer Inst.* 64:1091–1103.
14. Greenwald, P. and A. K. Polan. 1979. Lung cancer deaths among women. *New Eng. J. Med. 301*:274.
15. National Center for Health Statistics. 1978. *Health: United States, 1978.* Hyattsville, Maryland.
16. The thyroid gland is immediately adjacent to the thymus gland in the region where the neck joins the chest. Irradiation of the thymus inevitably results in irradiation of the thyroid gland. Hutchison, G. B. 1977. Carcinogenic effects of medical irradiation. In *Origins of Human Cancer,* pp. 501–509.
17. Hammond, E. C., L. Garfinkel, H. Seidman and E. A. Lew. 1977. Some recent findings concerning cigarette smoking. In *Origins of Human Cancer,* pp. 389–398.
18. Blot, W. J., T. J. Mason, R. Hoover and J. F. Fraumeni, Jr. 1977. Cancer by county: Etiologic implications. In *Origins of Human Cancer,* pp. 21–32.
19. Mason, T. J., R. Hoover, W. J. Blot and J. F. Fraumeni, Jr. 1975. *Atlas of Cancer Mortality for U.S. Counties: 1950–1969.* U.S. Department of Health, Education, and Welfare, Washington, D.C.
20. Doll, R. 1977. Introduction. In *Origins of Human Cancer,* pp. 1–12.
21. This analysis assumes no significant differences from country to country in inherited susceptibility to cancer (see Chapter 5). To a first approximation this is probably justified. It is difficult to imagine a genetic basis for even a 4-fold difference in the cancer rates in two large populations, let alone a 300-fold difference. For a more convincing argument against genetic differences, read on.
22. Hirayama, T. 1977. Changing patterns of cancer in Japan with special reference to the decrease in stomach cancer mortality. In *Origins of Human Cancer,* pp. 55–75.
23. Weisburger, J. H., L. A. Cohen and E. L. Wynder. 1977. On the etiology and metabolic epidemiology of the main human cancers. In *Origins of Human Cancer,* pp. 567–602. See also Haenszel, W. and M. Kurihara. 1968. Studies of Japanese migrants. I. Mortality from cancer and other diseases among Japanese in the United States. *J. Natl. Cancer Inst.* 40:43–68.
24. This figure is calculated from $1 - (1/\text{ratio of rates})$.
25. Berg, J. W. 1977. World-wide variations in cancer incidence as clues to cancer origins. In *Origins of Human Cancer,* pp. 15–19.
26. Based on data of Figure 10 and on a 1975 United States population estimated at 213,200,000 of which 51.3 percent were females.
27. The estimate is based on the fact that the five-year survival rate for all cancers is 40 percent. Many of those who survive five years after diagnosis of cancer eventually die of the disease, particularly in the case of such common cancers as those of the breast, colon, prostate, uterus, and lymphatic system. See also pp. 85–89 of Lewin, D. L., S. S. Devesa, J.

D. Godwin, II and D. T. Silverman. 1974. *Cancer Risks and Rates,* Second edition. U.S. Government Printing Office, Washington, D.C.

Chapter 2

1. An adult human has about 5 liters or 5×10^6 mm^3 of blood. Each mm^3 contains about 5×10^6 red blood cells (RBCs). Therefore, an adult contains $(5 \times 10^6) \times (5 \times 10^6) = 25 \times 10^{12}$ red blood cells. These 25×10^{12} red blood cells are completely replaced every 120 days (10^7 sec). Therefore, the turnover rate is $(25 \times 10^{12}$ RBC$)/10^7$ sec $= 2.5 \times 10^6$ cell divisions per second to maintain the right number of RBCs.
2. Photograph provided by C. Alex Shivers, University of Tennessee/BPS.
3. Photograph provided by Dr. Landrum B. Shettles, Las Vegas, Nevada.
4. Cells from many kinds of tissues, including cancer cells, can be grown in laboratory glassware, culture flasks, and dishes, in solutions that provide all the nutrients and other needed conditions (proper acidity and temperature, for example). Cultured cells can be grown attached to a clear surface so they can be conveniently observed with microscopes; or they can be grown suspended in nutrient solutions so they can be easily transferred or collected. Normal cells rarely survive for more than about 50 cell generations in artificial cultures. Cancer cells, by contrast, are generally long-lived, continuing to grow and reproduce indefinitely, long after the person from whom they were derived has died.
5. The arithmetic of such exponential growth is startling because the *rate* of increase speeds up. A single cell and all its descendants, dividing once a day for 30 days will form 2^{30} cells, i.e., just over one billion (10^9) cells. There would be twice as many cells one day later ($2 \times 2^{30} = 2^{31}$) and twice as many again the following day (2^{32}). By day 43, 2^{43} or 8.8 trillion cells will have formed. In the next day, an *additional* 8.8 trillion cells will form, resulting in more than 17 trillion cells in 44 days. This constantly accelerating *rate* of growth is one reason why it is so important to detect and treat cancers as early as possible, while they are small and growing relatively slowly. It is also the reason that even a single cancer cell that escapes treatment can reestablish the disease.
6. Photograph provided by Dr. P. P. H. DeBruyn and Dr. Y. Cho, Department of Anatomy, University of Chicago/BPS.
7. Additional details about the lymphatic system are available in most introductory biology texts and in Asimov, I. 1963. *The Human Body, Its Structure and Operation.* Mentor Books/New American Library, New York, and Jerne, N. K. 1963. The immune system. *Scientific American* 208:80–90.
8. Nicolson, G. L. 1979. Cancer metastasis. *Scientific American* 240:66–76; see also Nicolson, G. L. 1978. Experimental tumor metastasis. *Bioscience* 28:441–447; and Roos, E. and K. P. Dingemans. 1979. Mechanisms of metastasis. *Biochim. Biophys. Acta* 560:135–166.
9. See paper by G. L. Nicolson cited in Note 8.
10. Inagaki, J., V. Rodriguez and G. P. Bodey. 1974. Causes of death in cancer patients. *Cancer* 33:568–572.

11. Cancers of nerve cells are known, but these invariably occur during early postnatal development, when those nerve cells are still capable of dividing. Brain tumors arise from nonnerve cells of the brain, for example, glial cells. Such tumors are called gliomas.
12. Chapter 4 describes the chemistry of genes and the nature of mutations.

Chapter 3

1. Micrograph prepared with the generous cooperation of Dr. Louis Fink, Department of Pathology, University of Colorado Medical School.
2. The reader will find additional information about the structure and organization of cells in standard introductory biology texts such as Wilson, E. O., T. Eisner, W. R. Briggs, R. E. Dickerson, R. L. Metzenberg, R. D. O'Brien, M. Susman and W. E. Boggs. 1978. *Life on Earth,* Second edition. Sinauer Associates, Sunderland, Massachusetts; and Curtis, H. C. 1979. *Biology,* Third edition. Worth Publishers, New York.
3. Photograph provided by Professor David M. Prescott, University of Colorado, Boulder.
4. Photograph provided by Professor Keith R. Porter, University of Colorado, Boulder.
5. Photograph provided by Professor Keith R. Porter, University of Colorado, Boulder.
6. Photograph provided by Professor Keith R. Porter, University of Colorado, Boulder.
7. Photograph provided by Professor J. Richard McIntosh, University of Colorado, Boulder.
8. Micrographs of normal chromosomes provided by Dr. Arthur Robinson, National Jewish Hospital, Denver, Colorado. Micrograph of abnormal chromosomes provided by Dr. Avery A. Sandberg, Roswell Park Memorial Institute, Rochester, New York.
9. Photographs provided by Professor Walter S. Plaut, University of Wisconsin, Madison.
10. Prescott, D. M. 1977. *Reproduction of Eukaryotic Cells.* Academic Press, New York.

Chapter 4

1. Readers who wish to pursue this topic in additional depth may consult an introductory college-level biology text (for example, those listed in Note 2 for Chapter 3).
2. For an account of the evolution of this generalization, see Judson, H. F. 1979. *The Eighth Day of Creation.* Simon and Schuster, New York.

Chapter 5

1. Figure 5 in Chapter 2 is a reminder of how mutations may cause cancer.
2. Edwards, G. S. and J. G. Fox. 1979. Significance of nitrosamines in animal diets. *Science 203*:6.

3. Burridge, M. J., C. J. Wilcox and J. M. Hennemann. 1979. Influence of genetic factors on the susceptibility of cattle to bovine leukemia virus infection. *Europ. J. Cancer* 15:1395–1400.

4. Anders, A. and F. Anders. 1978. Etiology of cancer as studied in the platyfish–swordtail system. *Biochim. Biophys. Acta* 516:61–95. Professor Anders kindly provided the photographs in Figure 1. See also Gordon, M. 1959. The melanoma cell as an incompletely differentiated cell. In M. Gordon (ed.). *Pigment Cell Biology*. Academic Press, New York, pp. 215–239.

5. Gateff, E. 1978. Malignant neoplasms of genetic origin in *Drosophila melanogaster*. *Science* 200:1448–1459.

6. Fraumeni, J. F., Jr. 1977. Clinical patterns of familial cancer. In J. J. Mulvihill, R. W. Miller and J. F. Fraumeni, Jr. (eds.). *Progress in Cancer Research and Therapy, Vol. 3, Genetics of Human Cancer*. Raven Press, New York, pp. 223–233.

7. At a one-in-four overall rate, we expect about 24 percent of families of five to be cancer-free and about 40 percent of such families to sustain one cancer. Only about 16 of a thousand families of five are expected to include four or five cancer victims.

8. Knudson, A. G., Jr. 1977. Genetic and environmental interactions in the origin of human cancer. In *Progress in Cancer Research and Therapy*, cited in Note 6. See also Chapter 9.

9. Bolande, R. P. 1978. Childhood tumors and their relationship to birth defects. In *Progress in Cancer Research and Therapy*, cited in Note 6, pp. 43–75. See also Knudson, A. G., Jr. 1978. Retinoblastoma: A prototypic hereditary neoplasm. *Seminars in Oncology* 5:57–60.

10. Remember that the nucleus of each cell contains two sets of chromosomes (one from each parent) and thus two copies of each gene.

11. Germ cells are the reproductive cells that fuse during fertilization: egg and sperm. Mutated germ cells are formed either when a normal sperm or egg suffers a mutation or when a cell that produces germ cells suffers a mutation.

12. Hirayama, T. 1977. Changing patterns of cancer in Japan with special reference to the decrease in stomach cancer. In *Origins of Human Cancer*, pp. 55–75.

13. Henderson, B. E., M. C. Pike, V. R. Gerkins and J. T. Casagrande, 1977. The hormonal basis of breast cancer: Elevated plasma levels of estrogen, prolactin and progesterone. In *Origins of Human Cancer*, pp. 77–86.

14. Hutchison, G. B. 1977. Carcinogenic effects of medical irradiation. In *Origins of Human Cancer*, pp. 501–509.

15. Lynch, H. T., J. Lynch and P. Lynch. 1977. Management and control of familial cancer. In *Progress in Cancer Research and Therapy*, cited in Note 6, pp. 235–253.

16. See Figure 1, Chapter 1.

17. Approximately 13,600 new cases of melanoma are estimated to have occurred in the United States in 1979, out of a total of about 400,000 new skin cancer cases.

18. It is not conclusively known how ultraviolet light causes skin cancer; what is known is described in Chapter 8.

19. Hecht, F. and B. K. McCaw. 1977. Chromosome instability syndromes. In *Progress in Cancer Research and Therapy.* Cited in Note 6, pp. 107–123.

Chapter 6

1. Hill, J. 1761. Cautions against the immoderate use of snuff. Printed for R. Baldwin in Pater-noster Row and J. Jackson in St. James's Street, cited in Redmond, D. E., Jr. 1970. Tobacco and cancer: the first clinical report, 1761. *New Eng. J. Med. 282:*18–23.
2. Blot, W. J., T. J. Mason, R. Hoover and J. F. Fraumeni, Jr. 1977. Cancer by county: etiologic implications. In *Origins of Human Cancer,* pp. 29–32.
3. Pott, P. 1775. *Chirurgical Observations Relative to the Polypus of the Nose, the Cancer of the Scrotum, the Different Kinds of Ruptures, and the Mortification of the Toes and Feet.* Hawes, Clarke and Collins, London.
4. Lloyd, J. W. 1971. Long-term mortality study of steel workers. V. Respiratory cancer in coke plant workers. *J. Occup. Med. 13:*53–68.
5. U.S. Department of Health, Education, and Welfare. 1979. Smoking and Health: A Report of the Surgeon General. Washington, D.C.
6. IARC Working Group. 1980. Evaluations of chemicals and industrial processes associated with cancer in humans, based on human and animal data. *Cancer Res. 40:*1–12.
7. Doll, R. 1977. Introduction. In *Origins of Human Cancer,* pp. 2–12.
8. See for example Rinkus, S. J. and M. S. Legator. 1979. Chemical characterization of 465 known or suspected carcinogens and their correlation with mutagenic activity in the *Salmonella typhimurium* system. *Cancer Res. 39:*3289–3318. See also *Ca Selects—Carcinogens, Mutagens, and Teratogens,* published monthly by the National Cancer Institute, and distributed by the National Technical Information Service, Springfield, Virginia, for numerous abstracts of publications on carcinogens in animals.
9. Hernberg, S. 1977. Incidence of cancer in populations with exceptional exposure to metals. In *Origins of Human Cancer,* pp. 147–157.
10. Wilson, R. H., F. DeEds and A. J. Cox. 1941. The toxicity and carcinogenic activity of 2-acetylaminofluorene. *Cancer Res. 1:*595–608.
11. Wolfe, S. M. 1977. Standards for carcinogens: science affronted by politics. In *Origins of Human Cancer,* pp. 1735–1747.
12. See for example, Miller, J. A. and E. C. Miller. 1977. Ultimate chemical carcinogens as reactive mutagenic electrophiles. In *Origins of Human Cancer,* pp. 605–628.
13. McCann, J. and B. N. Ames. 1977. The *Salmonella*/microsome mutagenicity test: predictive value for animal carcinogenicity. In *Origins of Human Cancer,* pp. 1431–1450.
14. This important insight is thoroughly documented by papers in Section 9 of *Origins of Human Cancer,* pp. 605–726. See also DePierre, J. W. and L. Ernster. 1978. The metabolism of polycyclic hydrocarbons and its relationship to cancer. *Biochim. Biophys. Acta 473:*149–186.

15. The distribution of benzopyrenes in the environment can be assessed through the many sources indicated by the index in *Origins of Human Cancer,* p. 1863.
16. Jerina, D. M., R. Lehr, M. Schaefer-Ridder, H. Yagi, J. M. Karle, D. R. Thakker, A. W. Wood, A. Y. H. Lu, D. Ryan, S. West, W. Levin and A. H. Conney. 1977. Bay-region epoxides of dihydrodiols: a concept explaining the mutagenic and carcinogenic activity of benzo[*a*]pyrene and benz[*a*]anthracene. In *Origins of Human Cancer,* pp. 639–658.
17. See for example, Miller, R. W. 1977. Prenatal factors. In *Origins of Human Cancer,* pp. 381–388.
18. Meselson, M. and K. Russell. 1977. Comparisons of carcinogenic and mutagenic potency. In *Origins of Human Cancer,* pp. 1473–1481.
19. Higginson, J. 1969. Present trends in cancer epidemiology. In J. F. Morgan (ed.). *Proceedings of the Eighth Canadian Cancer Research Conference, 1968.* Pergamon Press, New York, pp. 40–75. See also Doll, R. 1977. Strategy for detection of cancer hazards to man. *Nature 265:*589–597.
20. This is an estimate based on numerous sources, for example, those cited in Notes 5, 9 and 15, and Tomatis, L. 1977. The value of long-term testing for the implementation of primary prevention. In *Origins of Human Cancer,* pp. 1339–1357. See also U. Saffiotti and J. K. Wagoner (eds.). 1976. *Occupational Carcinogenesis. Ann. N. Y. Acad. Sci.,* Vol. *271.*

Chapter 7

1. Pott, P. 1775. *Chirurgical Observations Relative to the Polypus of the Nose, the Cancer of the Scrotum, the Different Kinds of Ruptures, and the Mortification of the Toes and Feet.* Hawes, Clarke, and Collins, London, England.
2. Doll, R. 1977. Introduction. In *Origins of Human Cancer,* pp. 3–12.
3. IARC Working Group. 1980. An evaluation of chemicals and industrial processes associated with cancer in humans based on human and animal data. *Cancer Res. 40:* 1–12.
4. Yamagiwa, K. and K. Ichikawa. 1918. Experimentelle Studie über die Pathogenese der Epithelialgeschwulste. *Mitteilungen Med. Fakultät Kaiserl. Univ. Tokyo 15:* 295–344. See also Yamagiwa, K. and K. Ichikawa. 1918. Experimental study of the pathogenesis of carcinoma. *J. Cancer Res. 3:* 1.
5. Melick, W. F., J. J. Naryka and R. E. Kelly. 1971. Bladder cancer due to exposure to para-aminobiphenyl: a 17-year follow-up. *J. Urology 106:* 220–226.
6. Williams, M. H. C. 1958. Occupational tumours of the bladder. *Cancer 3:* 337–343.
7. U.S. Department of Health, Education, and Welfare. 1979. *Smoking and Health, a Report of the Surgeon General.* Washington, D.C.
8. Archer, V. E., J. D. Gillam and J. K. Wagoner. 1976. Respiratory disease mortality among uranium miners. In U. Saffiotti and J. K. Wagoner (eds.). *Occupational Carcinogenesis. Ann. N. Y. Acad. Sci. 271:* 280–293.

9. Selikoff, I. J., E. C. Hammond and J. Churg. 1968. Asbestos exposure, smoking and neoplasia. *J. Am. Med. Assoc. 204*: 104–110. See also Selikoff, I. J. 1977. Cancer risk of asbestos exposure. In *Origins of Human Cancer*, pp. 1765–1784.

10. Nicholson, W. J. 1977. Occupational and environmental standards for asbestos and their relation to human disease. In *Origins of Human Cancer*, pp. 1785–1796.

11. McCann, J. and B. N. Ames. 1977. The *Salmonella*/microsome mutagenicity test: predictive value for animal carcinogenicity. In *Origins of Human Cancer*, pp. 1431–1450.

12. Benjamin, B. 1979. Tobacco smoking in the world. *WHO Chronicle 33*: 94–97.

13. Sobel, R. 1978. *They Satisfy*. Anchor Press/Doubleday, Garden City, New York.

14. Hill, J. 1761. Cautions against the immoderate use of snuff. Printed for R. Baldwin in Pater-noster Row and J. Jackson in St. James's Street, cited in Redmond, D. E., Jr. 1970. Tobacco and cancer: the first clinical report, 1761. *New Eng. J. Med. 282*: 18–23.

15. von Soemmering, S. T. Quoted in Redmond, D. E., Jr. 1970. Tobacco and cancer: the first clinical report, 1761. *New Eng. J. Med. 282*: 18–23.

16. Data taken from Table 2 of Chapter 5 of *Smoking and Health*, cited in Note 7.

17. Silverberg, E. 1981. Cancer statistics, 1981. *Ca—A Cancer Journal for Clinicians 31*: 13–28.

18. Given that 38 percent of males who smoke die of lung cancer at a rate 12 times greater than the 62 percent of males who do not smoke,

$$\text{proportion of lung cancer} = \frac{(\text{deaths among smokers}) - (\text{deaths among nonsmokers})}{(\text{deaths among smokers}) + (\text{deaths among nonsmokers})}$$

$$= \frac{0.38(12) - 0.62(1)}{0.38(12) + 0.62(1)} = 0.76 \ (\text{or } 76\%)$$

19. Holt, P. G. and D. Keast. 1977. Environmentally induced changes in immunological function: acute and chronic effects of inhalation of tobacco smoke and other atmospheric contaminants in man and experimental animals. *Bacteriological Rev. 41*: 205–216. See also Section 10 of *Smoking and Health*, cited in Note 7.

20. Cohen, D., S. F. Arai and J. D. Brain. 1979. Smoking impairs long-term clearance from the lung. *Science 204*: 514–517.

21. Redrawn from Figure 3 of Chapter 5 of *Smoking and Health* (cited in Note 7).

22. Albert, R. E. and F. J. Burns. 1977. Carcinogenic atmospheric pollutants and the nature of low-level risks. In *Origins of Human Cancer*, pp. 289–292.

23. Lloyd, O. Ll. 1978. Respiratory-cancer clustering associated with localized industrial air pollution. *The Lancet*, February 11, 1978, pp. 318–320.

24. Selikoff, I. J. 1977. Cancer risk of asbestos exposure. In *Origins of Human Cancer*, pp. 1765–1784.

25. Harris, R. H., T. Page and N. A. Reiches. 1977. Carcinogenic hazards of organic chemicals in drinking water. In *Origins of Human Cancer,* pp. 309–330. See also Simmon, V. F., K. Kanhanen, K. Mortelmans and R. Tardiff. 1978. *Mutation Res. 53*: 262.

26. Hoover, R. N., F. W. McKay and J. F. Fraumeni, Jr. 1976. Fluoridated drinking water and the occurrence of cancer. *J. Natl. Cancer Inst. 57*: 757–768. See also Erickson, J. D. 1978. Mortality in cities with fluoridated water. *New Eng. J. Med. 298*: 1112–1116.

27. Bross, I. D. J. and J. Coombs. 1976. Early onset of oral cancer among women who drink and smoke. *Oncology 33*: 136–139.

28. Tuyns, A. J., G. Pèquignot and J. S. Abbatucci. 1979. Oesophageal cancer and alcohol consumption; importance of type of beverage. *Int. J. Cancer 23*: 443–447. See also Tuyns, A. J. 1979. Alcohol and cancer. *Cancer Res. 39*: 2840–2843.

29. Hinds, M. W., D. B. Thomas and H. P. O'Reilley. 1979. Asbestos, dental x-rays, tobacco, and alcohol in the epidemiology of laryngeal cancer. *Cancer 44*: 1114–1120.

30. See *Science 204*: 909 (1979) for references to tea and esophageal cancer.

31. Segi, M. 1975. Tea gruel as a possible factor for cancer of the esophagus. *Gann Japanese J. of Cancer Res. 66:* 199–202.

32. Kapadia, G. J., B. D. Paul, E. B. Chung, B. Ghosh and S. N. P. Radhan. 1976. Carcinogenicity of *Camellia sinensis* (Tea) and some tannin-containing folk medicinal herbs administered subcutaneously in rats. *J. Natl. Cancer Res. 57*: 207–209.

33. Timson, J. 1977. Caffeine. *Mutation Res. 47*: 1–52. See also MacMahon, B., S. Yen, D. Trichopoulos, K. Warren and G. Nardi. 1981. Coffee and cancer of the pancreas. *New Eng. J. Med. 304*: 630–633.

34. Miller, J. A. and E. C. Miller. 1977. Ultimate chemical carcinogens as reactive mutagenic electrophiles. In *Origins of Human Cancer,* pp. 605–627.

35. Doll, R. 1977. Strategy for detection of cancer hazards to man. *Nature 265*: 589–596. See also *Nature 256*: 540 for references to aflatoxins.

36. Kraybill, H. F. 1969. The toxicology and epidemiology of mycotoxins. *Tropical and Geographical Medicine 21*: 1–18.

37. Butler, W. H. 1964. Acute toxicity of aflatoxin B_1 in rats. *British J. Cancer 18*: 756–762. See also Wogan, G. N. and P. M. Newberne, 1967. Dose-response characteristics of aflatoxin B_1 carcinogenesis in the rat. *Cancer Res. 27*: 2370–2376.

38. Peers, F. G., G. A. Gilman and C. A. Linsell. 1976. Dietary aflatoxins and human liver cancer. A study in Swaziland. *Intl. J. Cancer 17*: 167–176.

39. For example, Lijinsky, W. and P. Shubik. 1964. Benzo[*a*]pyrene and other polynuclear hydrocarbons in charcoal-broiled meat. *Science 145*: 53–55. See also Lowenfels, A. B. and M. E. Anderson. 1977. Diet and cancer. *Cancer 39*: 1809–1814.

40. Commoner, B., A. J. Vithayathil, P. Dolara, S. Nair, P. Madyastha and G. C. Cuca. 1978. Formation of mutagens in beef and beef extract during cooking. *Science 201*: 913–916.

41. For a brief editorial review that contains an important list of references, consult Saccharin: from carcinogen to promoter, 1979. *Nature 278*: 123–124.

42. Clemmensen, J. 1977. Correlation of sites. In *Origins of Human Cancer,* pp. 87–100.

43. Mondall, S., D. W. Brankow and C. Heidelberger. 1978. Enhancement of oncogenesis in C3H/10T1/2 mouse embryo cell cultures by saccharin. *Science 201*: 1441–1442.

44. Lijinsky, W. and H. W. Taylor. 1977. Nitrosamines and their precursors in food. In *Origins of Human Cancer,* pp. 1579–1590.

45. Sen, N. P., W. F. Miles, B. Donaldson, T. Panalaks and J. R. Iyengar. 1973. Formation of nitrosamines in a meat curing mixture. *Nature 245*: 104–105. See also Fong, Y. Y. and W. C. Chan. 1973 Bacterial production of di-methyl nitrosamine in salted fish. *Nature 243*: 421–422.

46. Fine, D. H., D. P. Rounbehler, T. Fan and R. Ross. 1977. Human exposure to N-nitroso compounds in the environment. In *Origins of Human Cancer,* pp. 293–307. See also Gough, T. A. and C. L. Walters. 1978. Volatile nitrosamines in fried bacon. In *Some N-nitroso compounds,* IARC Monograph 17. IARC, Lyons, France, pp. 195–203.

47. Ho, J. H. C., D. P. Huang and Y. Y. Fong. 1978. Salted fish and nasopharyngeal carcinoma in Southern Chinese. *The Lancet,* September 16, 1978, pp. 626.

48. Tannenbaum, S. R., M. C. Archer, J. S. Wishnok, P. Correa, C. Cuello and W. Haenszel. 1977. Nitrate and the etiology of gastric cancer. In *Origins of Human Cancer,* pp. 1609–1625. See also Tannenbaum, S. R., D. Moran, W. Rand, C. Cuello and P. Correa. 1979. Gastric cancer in Colombia. IV. Nitrite and other ions in gastric contents of residents from a high risk region. *J. Natl. Cancer Inst. 62*:9–12.

49. Shirasu, Y., M. Moriya, K. Kato, F. Lienard, H. Tezuka and S.Teramoto. 1977. Mutagenicity screening on pesticides and modification products: A basis of carcinogenicity evaluation. In *Origins of Human Cancer,* pp. 267–285.

50. Armstrong, B. K. and R. Doll. 1975. Environmental factors and cancer incidence and the role of diet in human carcinogenesis with mortality in different countries with special reference to dietary practices. *Int. J. Cancer 15*: 617–631.

51. Weisburger, J. H., L. A. Cohen and E. L. Wynder. 1977. On the etiology and metabolic epidemiology of the main human cancers. In *Origins of Human Cancer,* pp. 567–602.

52. Graham, S., H. Dayal, M. Swanson, A. Mittleman and G. Williams, 1978. Diet in the epidemiology of cancer of the colon and rectum. *J. Natl. Cancer Inst. 61*: 709–714.

53. Hill, M. J. 1977. The role of unsaturated bile acids in the etiology of large bowel cancer. In *Origins of Human Cancer,* pp. 1627–1640. See also Lowenfels, A. B. 1968. Does bile promote extra-colonic cancer? *The Lancet,* July 29, 1978, pp. 239–241.

54. Williams, R. R., N. L. Stegens and J. R. Goldsmith. 1977. Associations of cancer site and type with occupation and industry from the Third National Cancer Survey interview. *J. Natl. Cancer Inst. 59*: 1147–1185. See also Schottenfeld, D. and J. F. Haas. 1979. Carcinogens in the workplace. *Ca—A Cancer Journal for Clinicians 29*: 144–168.

55. Monson, R. R. and L. J. Fine. 1978. Cancer mortality and morbidity among rubber workers. *J. Natl. Cancer Inst. 61*: 1047–1053. See also Fajen, J. M., G. A. Carson, D. P. Rounbehler, T. Y. Fan, R. Vita, U. E.

Goff, M. H. Wolf, G. S. Edwards, D. H. Fine, V. Reinhold and K. Bieman. 1979. *N*-Nitrosamines in the rubber and tire industry. *Science* 205: 1262–1264.

56. Ammenheuser M.M. and M. E. Warren. 1979. Detection of mutagens in the urine of rats following topical application of hair dyes. *Mutation Res.* 66: 241–245. See also Nasca, P. C., C. E. Lawrence, P. Greenwald, S. Chorost, J. T. Arbuckle and A. Paulson, 1980. Relationship of hair dye use, benign breast disease, and breast cancer. *J. Natl. Cancer Inst.* 64: 23–28.

57. Menck, H. R., M. C. Pike, B. E. Henderson and J. S. Jing. 1977. Lung cancer risk among beauticians and other female workers. *J. Natl. Cancer Inst.* 59: 1423–1425.

58. See Note 2 and also Jick, H. and P. G. Smith. 1977. Regularly used drugs and cancer. In *Origins of Human Cancer,* pp. 389–398.

59. Fraumeni, J. F., Jr. 1979. Epidemiological studies of cancer. In A. C. Griffin and C. R. Shaw (eds.). *Carcinogens: Identification and Mechanisms of Action.* Raven Press, New York, pp. 51–63. See also Tomatis, L., C. Agthe, H. Bartsch, J. Huff, R. Montesano, R. Saracci, E. Walker and J. Wilbourn. 1978. Evaluation of the carcinogenicity of chemicals: A review of the monograph program of the International Agency for Research on Cancer (1971–1977). *Cancer Res.* 38: 877–885.

60. Williams, R. R., M. Feinleib, R. J. Conner and N. L. Stegens. 1978. Case-control study of antihypertensive and diuretic use by women with malignant and benign breast lesions detected in a mammography screening program. *J. Natl. Cancer Inst.* 61: 327–335.

61. Schmahl, D., R. Port and J. Wahrendorf. 1977. A dose-response study on urethane carcinogenesis in rats and mice. *Intl. J. Cancer* 19: 77–80. See also Tomatis, L. 1977. The value of long-term testing for implementation of primary prevention. In *Origins of Human Cancer,* pp. 1347–1357.

62. Tomatis, L. 1977. Cited in Note 61.

63. Hoover, R., L. A. Gray, Sr. and J. F. Fraumeni, Jr. 1977. Stilbestrol (diethylstilbestrol), and the risk of ovarian cancer. *The Lancet,* September 10, 1977 (pp. 533–534). See also Tomatis, L. 1977. Cited in Note 61.

64. Brackbill, Y. and H. W. Berendes. 1978. Dangers of diethylstilbestrol: Review of a 1953 paper. *The Lancet,* September 2, 1978, p. 520.

65. Antunes, C. M. F., P. D. Stolley, N. B. Rosenshein, J. L. Davies, J. A. Tonascia, C. Brown, L. Burnett, A. Rutledge, M. Pokempner and R. Garcia. 1979. Endometrial cancer and estrogen use. Report of a large case-control study. *New Eng. J. Med.* 300: 9–13.

66. Blum, A. and B. N. Ames. 1976. Flame-retardant additives as possible cancer hazards. *Science* 195: 17–23.

67. Benditt, E. P. 1977. The origin of atherosclerosis. *Scientific American* 236: 74–85.

Chapter 8

1. Ujeno, Y. 1978. Carcinogenic hazard from natural background radiation in Japan. *J. Radiation Res.* 19: 205–212.

2. Liebeskind, D., R. Bases, F. Mendez, F. Elequin and M. Koenigsberg.

1979. Sister chromatid exchanges in human lymphocytes after exposure to diagnostic ultrasound. *Science 205*: 1273–1275.

3. Clemmesen, J. 1977. Correlation of sites. In *Origins of Human Cancer*, pp. 87–100.

4. Silverberg, E. 1981. Cancer statistics, 1981. *Ca—A Cancer Journal for Clinicians 31*: 13–28.

5. For review and references, see Kripke, M. L. 1979. Speculations on the role of ultraviolet radiation in the development of malignant melanoma. *J. Natl. Cancer Inst. 63*: 541–548.

6. Viola, M. W. 1979. Solar cycles and malignant melanoma. *Medical Hypotheses 5*: 153–160.

7. Smith, T. 1979. The Queensland melanoma project. *British Medical Journal 1*: 253–254.

8. Ackerknecht, E. H. 1972. *History and Geography of the Most Important Diseases*. Hafner, New York.

9. Dublin, L. I. and M. Spiegelmann. 1947. The longevity and mortality of American physicians, 1938–1942. *J. Am. Med. Assoc. 134*: 1211–1215.

10. Upton, A. C. 1977. Radiation effects. In *Origins of Human Cancer*, pp. 477–500.

11. Weiss, W. 1979. Changing incidence of thyroid cancer. *J. Natl. Cancer Inst. 62*: 1137–1142.

12. Hutchison, G. B. 1977. Carcinogenic effects of medical irradiation. In *Origins of Human Cancer*, pp. 501–509.

13. Polednak, A. P. 1978. Bone cancer among female radium dial workers. Latency periods and incidence rates by time after exposure. *J. Natl. Cancer Inst. 60*: 77–82.

14. Dickson, D. 1977. Doctors claim A-bomb tests linked to rise in child leukemia deaths. *Nature 277*: 420.

15. Martell, E. A. 1975. Tobacco, radioactivity, and cancer in smokers. *American Scientist 63*: 404–412.

16. Photographs provided by Dr. Arthur Robinson, National Jewish Hospital, Denver, Colorado.

17. Najarian, T. and T. Colton. 1978. Mortality from leukemia and cancer in shipyard nuclear workers. *The Lancet*, May 13, 1978, pp. 1018–1020.

18. See reviews by Marx, J. L. 1979. Low-level radiation: just how bad is it? *Science 204*: 160–164. See also Savage, J. R. K. 1979. Chromosomal aberrations at very low radiation doses. *Nature 277*: 512–513.

Chapter 9

1. Ellermann, V. and O. Bang. 1908. Experimentelle Leukämie bei Hühnern. *Zentralbl. Bacteriol.*, Abt. I 46:595. See also Ellermann, V. and O. Bang. 1909. Experimentelle Leukämie bei Hühnern. *Z. Hyg. Infekt. 63*: 231.

2. These criteria are usually called KOCH'S POSTULATES after the nineteenth century bacteriologist who formulated them.

3. For an introduction to viruses see any introductory biology text, for example, by Wilson, E. O. and others. 1978. *Life on Earth*, Second edition. Sinauer Associates, Sunderland, Massachusetts.

4. Micrograph provided by Professor Harald zur Hausen, Institute for Virology in the Center for Hygiene and the Clinic of the Albert Ludwigs University, Freiburg im Breisgau, Federal Republic of Germany.

5. Tooze, J. (ed.). *The Molecular Biology of Tumour Viruses.* Cold Spring Harbor Laboratory, Cold Spring Harbor, New York. 1973.

6. Rapp, F. and C. L. Reed. 1977. The viral etiology of cancer. *Cancer 40*: 419–429. See also Major, E. O., M. Fiori, G. di Mayorca and C. Zacharias. 1977. BK, a human polyoma virus—its biology, biochemistry, and association with human tumors. *Origins of Human Cancer,* pp. 989–1007.

7. Orth, G., F. Breitburd, M. Favre and O. Croissant. 1977. Papillomaviruses: possible role in human cancers. In *Origins of Human Cancer,* pp. 1043–1068.

8. *The Molecular Biology of Tumour Viruses.* Cited in Note 5, pp. 38–39.

9. Photograph provided by Dr. J. T. Finch, Cambridge, England.

10. *The Molecular Biology of Tumour Viruses.* Cited in Note 5, p. 42.

11. *The Molecular Biology of Tumour Viruses.* Cited in Note 5, p. 421. See also Fenner, F., B. R. McAuslan, C. A. Mims, J. Sambrook and D. O. White. 1974. *The Biology of Animal Viruses,* Second edition. Academic Press, New York, pp. 352–358.

12. *The Molecular Biology of Tumour Viruses.* Cited in Note 5, pp. 477–485.

13. Nazerian, K. and R. L. Witter. 1970. Cell-free transmission and *in vivo* replication of Marek's disease virus. *J. Virol. 5*:388–397. See also Nazerian, K. 1979. Marek's disease lymphoma of chicken and its causative herpesvirus. *Biochim. Biophys. Acta 560*: 375–395.

14. Rapp, F. 1978. Herpesviruses, venereal disease, and cancer. *Am. Scientist* 66: 670–674.

15. *The Molecular Biology of Tumour Viruses.* Cited in Note 5, Chapter 11.

16. Photograph provided by Professor Etienne de Harven of the Memorial Sloan-Kettering Cancer Center.

17. *The Molecular Biology of Tumour Viruses.* Cited in Note 5, pp. 30–34.

18. Photograph provided by Dr. Dorothy R. Pitelka, Cancer Research Laboratory, University of California, Berkeley.

19. McGrath, C. M. and H. D. Soule. 1977. An inquiry into the involvement of nonhuman breast cancer viruses in human disease: virus expression in malignant breast ductal stem cells. In *Origins of Human Cancer,* pp. 1287–1303. See also Ohno, T., R. Mesa-Tejada, I. Keydar, M. Ramanarayanan, J. Bausch and S. Spiegelman. 1979. Human breast carcinoma antigen is immunologically related to the polypeptide of the group-specific glycoprotein of mouse mammary tumor virus. *Proc. Natl. Acad. Sci.* (US) 76: 2460–2464. See also Kantor, J. A., Y-H. Lee, J. G. Chirikjian and W. F. Feller. 1979. DNA polymerase with characteristics of reverse transcriptase purified from human milk. *Science 204*: 511–513.

20. Gross, L. 1951. "Spontaneous" leukemia developing in C3H mice following inoculation, in infancy, with AK-leukemic extracts, or AK embryos. *Proc. Soc. Exp. Biol. Med.* 76: 27–32.

21. For example, Gunz, F. W., J. P. Gunz, P. C. Vincent, M. Bergin, F. L. Johnson, H. Bashir and R. L. Kirk. 1978. Thirteen cases of leukemia in a family. *J. Natl. Cancer Inst.* 60: 1243–1250.

22. Essex, M., S. M. Cotter, J. R. Stephenson, S. A. Aaronson and W. D.

Hardy, Jr. 1977. Leukemia, lymphoma, and fibrosarcoma of cats as models for similar diseases of man. In *Origins of Human Cancer,* pp. 1197–1214.

23. Jarrett, W. F. H. 1977. The development of vaccines against feline leukemia. In *Origins of Human Cancer,* pp. 1215–1222.

24. Tegtmeyer, P. and K. Rundell. 1977. The role of the papovavirus gene A in oncogenic transformation. In *Origins of Human Cancer,* pp. 957–969.

25. *The Molecular Biology of Tumour Viruses.* Cited in Note 5, pp. 590–602.

26. Gardner, M. B., S. Rashad, S. Shimizu, R. W. Rongey, B. E. Henderson, R. M. McAllister, V. Klement, H. P. Charman, R. V. Gilden, R. L. Heberling and R. J. Huebner. 1977. Search for RNA tumor virus in humans. In *Origins of Human Cancer,* pp. 1235–1252. See also Gallo, R. C., W. C. Saxinger, R. E. Gallagher, D. H. Gillespie, G. S. Aulakh, F. Wong-Staal, F. Ruscetti and M. S. Reitz. 1977. Some ideas on the origin of leukemia in man and recent evidence for the presence of type-C viral-related information. In *Origins of Human Cancer,* pp. 1253–1286.

27. Das, M. R., L. Padhy, R. Koshy, S. M. Sirsat and M. A. Rich. 1976. Human milk samples from different ethnic groups contain RNase that inhibits, and plasma membrane that stimulates reverse transcriptase. *Nature 262*: 802–805. See also Henderson, B. 1974. Type B virus and human breast cancer. *Cancer 34*: 1386. See also references listed under Note 22.

28. Kantor, J. A., Y-H. Lee, J. G. Chirikjian and W. F. Feller. 1979. DNA polymerase with characteristics of reverse transcriptase purified from human milk. *Science 204*: 511–513.

29. Rawls, W. E. and E. Adam. 1977. Herpes simplex viruses and human malignancies. In *Origins of Human Cancer,* pp. 1133–1155. See also Note 19.

30. Graham, S., R. Priore, M. Graham, R. Browne, W. Burnett and D. West. 1979. Genital cancer in wives of penile cancer patients. *Cancer 44*: 1870–1874.

31. de-Thé, G. 1977. Viruses as causes of some human tumors? Results and prospectives of the epidemiologic approach. In *Origins of Human Cancer,* pp. 1113–1131.

32. Henle, W., G. Henle and E. T. Lennette. 1979. The Epstein-Barr virus. *Scientific American 241*: 48–59.

Chapter 10

1. Silverberg, E. 1981. Cancer statistics, 1981. *Ca—A Cancer Journal for Clinicians 31*: 13–28. This figure excludes skin cancers: melanoma skin cancers are very malignant and metastasize rapidly; nonmelanoma skin cancers are not very malignant and are easily cured.

2. This estimate is made from data in Levin, D. L., S. S. Devesa, J. D. Godwin and D. T. Silverman. 1974. *Cancer Rates and Risks,* Second edition. U. S. Department of Health, Education and Welfare, Washington, D.C.

3. Prager, M. D. 1978. Specific cancer immunotherapy. *Cancer Immunol.*

Immunother. 3: 157–161. See also W. D. Terry and D. Windhorst (eds.). 1978. *Progress in Cancer Research and Therapy, Vol. 6, Immunotherapy of Cancer: Present Status of Trials in Man.* Raven Press, New York.

4. Pack, G. T. and I. M. Ariel. 1968. The history of cancer therapy. In *Cancer Management.* American Cancer Society, Lippincott, Philadelphia.

5. Adamson, R. H. and S. M. Sieber. 1977. Antineoplastic agents as potential carcinogens. *Origins of Human Cancer,* pp. 429–443.

6. Nemoto, T., J. Vana, R. N. Bedwani, H. W. Baker, F. H. McGregor and G. P. Murphy. 1980. Management and survival of female breast cancer: results of a national survey by the American College of Surgeons. *Cancer 45*: 2917–2924.

7. Simon, N. 1977. Breast cancer induced by radiation. Relation to mammography and treatment of acne. *J. Am. Med. Assoc. 237*: 789–790.

8. Stutman, O. 1977. Immunological surveillance. In *Origins of Human Cancer,* pp. 729–750.

9. Everson, T. C. and W. H. Cole. 1966. *Spontaneous Regression in Cancer.* W. B. Saunders Co., Philadelphia. See also Foulds, L. 1969. *Neoplastic Development.* Academic Press, London and New York.

10. U.S. Department of Health, Education, and Welfare, 1979. *Smoking and Health, a Report of the Surgeon General.* Washington, D. C., Sections 6 and 10.

11. Burke, D. C. 1977. The status of interferon. *Scientific American 236*: 42–50.

12. Fleckenstein, B. 1979. Oncogenic herpesviruses of non-human primates. *Biochim. Biophys. Acta 560*: 301–342.

13. A new technique for making specific anti-cancer antibodies has been developed by fusing lymphocytes with transformed cells (Chapter 9). The resulting hybrid cells (hybridomas) grow in culture and produce large amounts of monoclonal antibodies. These antibodies are directed against the cancer cells against which the original lymphocytes had been producing antibodies. Treatments using monoclonal antibodies have been successfully tested in animals but tests with humans have not begun.

Chapter 11

1. Pott, P. 1775. *Chirurgical Observations Relative to the Polypus of the Nose, the Cancer of the Scrotum, the Different Kinds of Ruptures, and the Mortification of the Toes and Feet.* Hawes, Clarke, and Collins, London.

2. Nachtwey, D. S. and R. D. Rundel. 1981. A photobiological evaluation of tanning booths. *Science 211*: 405–407.

3. Sontag, J., N. Page and U. Saffiotti. 1976. *Guidelines for Carcinogen Assay in Small Rodents.* Department of Health, Education, and Welfare, Washington, D.C.

4. Epstein, S. S. 1978. *The Politics of Cancer.* Sierra Club Books, San Francisco, p. 1.

5. Russell, M. A. H. 1971. Cigarette smoking: natural history of a dependence disorder. *Brit. J. Med. Psychol. 44*: 1–16.

6. See for example, Wolfe, S. M. 1977. Standards for carcinogens: science affronted by politics. In *Origins of Human Cancer,* pp. 1735–1747.

Chapter 12

1. Haagensen, C. D., E. Cooley, C. S. Kennedy, E. Miller, R. S. Handley, A. C. Thackray, H. R. Butcher, Jr., E. Dahl-Iversen, T. Tobiassen, I. G. Williams, M. P. Curwen, S. Kaae, and H. Johansen. 1963. Treatment of early mammary carcinoma. *Annals of Surgery 157:* 157.
2. For example, an easily understood booklet on how to examine one's breasts for suspicious lumps is available from the American Cancer Society as "How To Examine Your Breasts." The appendix to this book tells how to obtain this and other helpful publications.
3. Silverberg, E. 1981. Cancer statistics, 1981. *Ca—A Cancer Journal for Clinicians 31: 13–28.* (The data quoted are for 1965–1969. Differences between these data and those cited in Note 6 for Chapter 10 reflect differences in methods of collecting and reporting.)
4. Green, L. W. 1976. Site- and symptom-related factors in secondary prevention of cancer. In J. W. Cullen, B. H. Fox, and R. N. Isom (eds.). *Cancer: The Behavioral Dimensions.* Raven Press, New York,* pp. 45–61.
5. Enelow, A. J. 1976. Group influences on health behavior: a social learning perspective. In *Cancer: The Behavioral Dimensions,* pp. 63–73.
6. Holland, J. 1973. Psychologic aspects of cancer. In J. Holland and E. Frei, III (eds.). *Cancer Medicine.* Lea and Feibiger, Philadelphia, Pennsylvania, pp. 991–1021.
7. U.S. Department of Health and Human Services. 1980. *Coping with Cancer,* Washington, D.C.
8. Kutner, B. and G. Gordon, 1961. Seeking care for cancer. *J. Health and Human Behavior 2:* 171–178.
9. Henderson, J. G., E. D. Wittkower, and M. N. Lougheed. 1958. A psychiatric investigation of the delay factor in patient to doctor presentation in cancer. *J. Psychosomatic Res. 3:27–41.*
10. Kegeles, S. S. 1976. Relationship of sociocultural factors to cancer. In *Cancer: The Behavioral Dimensions,* pp. 101–109.
11. Oken, D. 1961. What to tell cancer patients: a study of medical attitudes. *J. Amer. Med. Assoc. 175:* 86–94.
12. Kelly, W. D. and S. R. Friesen. 1950. Do cancer patients want to be told? *Surgery 27:* 822–826.
13. Holland, J. 1980. Understanding the cancer patient. *Ca—A Cancer Journal for Clinicians 30:* 103–112.
14. Waxenberg, S. E. 1966. The importance of the communication of feelings about cancer. *Ann. N.Y. Acad. Sci. 125:* 1000–1005.
15. Vettese, J. M. 1976. Problems of the patient confronting the diagnosis of cancer. In *Cancer: The Behavioral Dimensions,* pp. 275–282.
16. Holland, J. 1976. Coping with cancer: a challenge to the behavioral sciences. In *Cancer: The Behavioral Dimensions,* pp. 263–268.
17. Peteet, J. R. 1979. Depression in cancer patients: an approach to differential diagnosis and treatment. *J. Amer. Med. Assoc. 241:* 1487–1489.

* In subsequent citations, this book will be referred to as *Cancer: The Behavioral Dimensions*.

18. Giacquinta, B. 1977. Helping families face the crisis of cancer. *Amer. J. Nursing* 77: 1585–1588.
19. Manos, J. J. 1980. Surviving cancer: the adaptation of the children of cancer victims. Unpublished Master's Thesis, University of California, Los Angeles.
20. Luce, J. K. and J. J. Dawson. 1975. Quality of life. *Seminars in Oncology* 2: 323–327.
21. Weisman, A. D. 1976. Coping behavior and suicide in cancer. In *Cancer: The Behavioral Dimensions,* pp. 331–341.
22. Several informative pamphlets on cancer of the larynx and laryngectomy rehabilitation are available from the American Cancer Society. (See the appendix to this book.)
23. Derogatis, L. R. and S. M. Kourlesis. 1981. An approach to evaluation of sexual problems in the cancer patient. *Ca—A Cancer Journal for Clinicians* 31: 46–50.
24. For more information on the job rights of cancer victims, a pamphlet entitled "If you Have Had Cancer—The Law Protects Your Job Rights" is available through the American Cancer Society. (See the appendix to this book.)
25. These data are taken from a study of 115 advanced cancer patients, published in 1973 by Cancer Care, Inc. of the National Cancer Fund under the title "Impact, costs, and consequences of catastrophic illnesses on patients and families."
26. Farberow, N., S. Gayles, F. Cutter, and D. Renolds. 1971. An eight-year survey of hospital suicides. *Life-Threatening Behavior* 1: 181–202. Also see Note 21.
27. Charmaz, K. 1980. *The Social Reality of Death.* Addison-Wesley, Reading, Massachusetts.
28. Hackett, T. 1976. Psychological assistance for the dying patient and his family. In R. E. Caughill (ed.). *The Dying Patient: A Supportive Approach.* Little, Brown and Company, Boston, Massachusetts, pp. 371–378.
29. Semipopular books that explore these topics include Caughill, R. E. 1976. *The Dying Patient: A Supportive Approach.* Addison-Wesley, Reading, Massachusetts, and Kubler-Ross, E. 1969. *On Death and Dying.* Macmillan, New York.
30. Schulz, R. 1978. *The Psychology of Death, Dying, and Bereavement.* Addison-Wesley, Reading, Massachusetts.
31. Bugen, L. A. 1979. Fundamentals of bereavement. In L. A. Bugen (ed.). *Death and Dying.* W. C. Brown, Dubuque, Iowa.
32. Holleb, A. I. 1974. A patient's right to die . . . The easy way out. *Ca—A Cancer Journal for Clinicians 24*: 256. Also see Notes 29 and 30.

Appendix

Cancer-Related Services and Resources

The following lists of services and resources provide the interested reader with starting points in the search for reliable information about various forms of cancer and for groups that assist cancer families in their struggles with the disease. These lists are not comprehensive but are as current as the printed medium permits.

Services of the National Cancer Institute

The National Cancer Institute (NCI) is a division of the National Institutes of Health. NCI supports major programs of basic research on the biology of cancer and related subjects as well as programs of basic and applied research directed toward developing and evaluating new treatments for cancer. NCI also supports the Office of Cancer Communications which administers the Cancer Information Service and provides other information services to the general public and the health care community.

CANCER INFORMATION SERVICE

The Cancer Information Service (CIS) is a national system of offices that can be reached by toll-free telephone numbers. Each office is staffed by specially trained volunteers and professionals who provide up to date information about the causes, prevention, detection, diagnosis, and treatment of the disease. Information is also available about the emotional aspects of cancer, about local cancer care facilities and support groups, and about rehabilitation programs for patients. The information specialists at the CIS offices provide this information in clear and easily understood language. CIS personnel also will send, upon the caller's request, free copies of pamphlets about particular forms of the disease, treatments and possible side effects, and nutritional information and recipes for the cancer patient. These pamphlets (listed below) are technically correct, yet written in clear and simple language; they will help the patient's family and friends as well as the patient.

STATE AND REGIONAL OFFICES OF THE CANCER
INFORMATION SERVICE

State and regional CIS offices, many of which are associated with Comprehensive Cancer Centers (listed below) are generally staffed only during local business hours. The national CIS telephone number, 1-800-638-6694, is staffed every day of the year, holidays included, from 8 A.M. to midnight, Eastern Time and may be called when services are not available from local CIS offices.

National

To be used in all states not served by regional offices; all states outside local business hours.

Office of Cancer Communications
National Cancer Institute
Building 31, Room 10A18
Bethesda, Maryland 20205
    1-800-638-6694

Alabama

Alabama Cancer Information Service
2160 Greensprings Highway
Birmingham, Alabama 35205
    1-800-292-6201

Alaska

Use National Cancer Institute address
    1-800-638-6070

California

LAC-USC Cancer Center
1721 Griffin Avenue
Los Angeles, California 90031

From Area Codes (213), (714) and (805):
    1-800-252-9066;
in other areas of the state, call
    (213) 226-2374

Connecticut

Yale Comprehensive Cancer Center
850 Howard Avenue
New Haven, Connecticut 06519
    1-800-922-0824

Delaware

Use Pennsylvania Address
    1-800-523-3586

District of Columbia

Howard University Cancer Center
2041 Georgia Avenue, N.W.
Room 301
Washington, D.C. 20060
Also for suburban Maryland and Northern Virginia
    (202) 636-5700

Florida

Comprehensive Cancer Center for the
State of Florida
P.O. Box 016960, D8-4
Miami, Florida 33101
1-800-432-5953
Spanish-speaking callers dial
1-800-432-5955
In Dade County, call
(305) 547-6920
Spanish-speaking callers dial
(305) 547-6960

Georgia

Use Florida Address
1-800-327-7332

Hawaii

Community Cancer Program of Hawaii
1236 Lauhala Street
Honolulu, Hawaii 96813
From Oahu, dial
536-0111
From neighboring islands, ask operator
for:
Enterprise 6702

Illinois

Illinois Cancer Council
36 South Wabash Avenue
Chicago, Illinois 60603
800-972-0586
In Chicago, call
(312) 226-2371

Kentucky

McDowell Community Cancer Network
915 South Limestone Street
Lexington, Kentucky 40536
800-432-9321

Maine

Maine Cancer Information Service
P.O. Box 8648
Portland, Maine 04104
1-800-225-7034

Maryland

The Johns Hopkins Office of Cancer
Communications
550 North Broadway
Baltimore, Maryland 21205
800-492-1444
For Metropolitan Washington, use
District of Columbia address
(202) 636-5700

Massachusetts

Sidney Farber Cancer Institute
44 Binney Street
Boston, Massachusetts 02115
1-800-952-7420

Michigan

Michigan Cancer Foundation
110 East Warren Street
Detroit, Michigan 48201
From (313) only:
800-462-9191

Minnesota

Mayo Comprehensive Cancer Center
Mayo Clinic and Foundation
200 S.W. First Street
Rochester, Minnesota 55901
1-800-582-5262

New Hampshire

New Hampshire Cancer Information
Service
22 Bridge Street
Manchester, New Hampshire 03101
1-800-225-7034

New Jersey (Northern)

Use New York City Address
800-223-1000

New Jersey (Southern)

Use Pennsylvania Address
800-523-3586

New York

For New York City: Memorial Sloan-
  Kettering Cancer Center
1275 York Avenue
New York, New York 10021
  (212) 794-7982
All other residents:
Roswell Park Memorial Institute
666 Elm Street
Buffalo, New York 14263
  1-800-462-7255

North Carolina

Duke Comprehensive Cancer Center
P.O. Box 2985
Durham, North Carolina 27710
  1-800-672-0943
In Durham County, call
  (919) 684-2230

North Dakota

Use Minnesota Address
  1-800-328-5188

Ohio

Ohio State University Comprehensive
  Cancer Center
101A Hamilton Hall
1645 Neil Avenue
Columbus, Ohio 43210
  1-800-282-6522

Pennsylvania

Fox Chase Cancer Center
7701 Burholme Avenue
Philadelphia, Pennsylvania 19111
  1-800-822-3963
Delaware (add 1-) and Southern New
  Jersey:
  800-523-3586

South Dakota

Use Minnesota Address
  1-800-328-5188

Texas

Cancer Information Service of Texas
The University of Texas System Cancer
  Center
M.D. Anderson Hospital and Tumor
  Institute
PR-920
Houston, Texas 77030
  1-800-392-2040
In Houston, call
  (713) 792-3245

Vermont

Vermont Cancer Information Service
1 South Prospect
Burlington, Vermont 05401
  1-800-225-7034

Virginia

American Cancer Society
Cancer Answer Service
In Richmond call:
  (804) 359-1308
Rest of Virginia:
  1-800-552-7996

Washington

Fred Hutchinson Cancer Research
  Center
1124 Columbia Street
Seattle, Washington 98104
  1-800-552-7212

Wisconsin

Wisconsin Clinical Cancer Center
1900 University Avenue
Madison, Wisconsin 53705
  1-800-362-8038

PUBLICATIONS OF THE OFFICE OF CANCER
COMMUNICATIONS/NATIONAL CANCER INSTITUTE
(PARTIAL LISTING)

General Materials

Asbestos Exposure: What it Means, What to Do

Breast Exams: What You Should Know

Breast Self-Examination

Cancer Treatment: "Medicine for the Layman" Series

Clearing the Air: A Guide to Quitting Smoking

Despejando El Aire: Guia Para Dejar De Fumar

Did You as a Child or a Young Adult Have X-ray Treatments Involving Your Head or Neck?

Everything Doesn't Cause Cancer

If You've Thought About Breast Cancer

Lo Que Usted Debe Saber Sobre El Cancer

Progress Against Breast Cancer, What You Can Do About It (Black Family Focus)

Progreso Contra El Cancer Del Seno, Lo Que Usted Puede Hacer

Progress Against . . . Series:
   Cancer of the Bladder
   Cancer of the Colon and Rectum
   Hodgkin's Disease
   Cancer of the Larynx
   Cancer of the Prostate
   Cancer of the Skin
   Cancer of the Stomach
   Cancer of the Testis
   Cancer of the Uterus
   Leukemias, Lymphomas & Multiple Myeloma

Progress Against Leukemia

Research Report: Cancer of the Lung

Science and Cancer

Were You or Your Daughter or Son Born After 1940?

What Black Americans Should Know About Cancer

Patient Materials

Chemotherapy and You: A Guide to Self-Help During Treatment

Diet and Nutrition: A Resource for Parents of Children with Cancer

Eating Hints: Recipes and Tips for Better Nutrition During Cancer Treatment

Hospital Days, Treatment Ways

The Leukemic Child

Questions and Answers about DES Exposure During Pregnancy and Before Birth

Radiation Therapy and You: A Guide to Self-Help During Treatment

Taking Time: Support for People with Cancer and the People Who Care About Them

What You Need to Know About Cancer . . . Series:
   Cancer (general)
   Bladder
   Bone
   Breast
   Colon and Rectum
   Dysplasia, Very Early Cancer and Invasive Cancer of the Cervix
   Esophagus
   Hodgkin's Disease
   Kidney
   Adult Leukemia
   Childhood Leukemia
   Lung
   Melanoma
   Mouth
   Multiple Myeloma
   Non-Hodgkin's Lymphoma
   Ovary
   Prostate
   Skin
   Stomach
   Uterus

Services of the American Cancer Society

The American Cancer Society (ACS) is a national voluntary organization that develops resources for programs of education, patient services, and rehabilitation. These programs, implemented by local ACS units in many communities across the country, include general information for cancer patients and their families (e.g., the publications listed below), counseling and guidance, and referrals to community health services and other local resources. The services available through local units vary from community to community, but may also include loans of equipment for the care of homebound patients, transportation to and from treatments, and rehabilitation programs.

The functional unit of the ACS is the local chapter. To locate the nearest local chapter, consult a local telephone directory or the nearest regional office (listed below). Four national programs sponsored by or associated with the ACS merit special mention.

Reach to Recovery. This organization attempts to meet the physical, emotional, and cosmetic needs of women who have undergone mastectomies. Referred by the patient's physician, carefully trained volunteers who have successfully adjusted to their own mastectomies visit new mastectomy patients. These volunteers bring information about rehabilitation exercises (the origin of the organization's name) and about prostheses and other cosmetic aids. Perhaps most importantly, they provide direct evidence that recovery from a mastectomy is possible. Reach to Recovery also supplies educational material to health professionals, including demonstrations and lectures at health care institutions.

International Association of Laryngectomies. Devoted to education and rehabilitation, the Association acts as an umbrella organization for more than 250 local clubs that support the full rehabilitation of people who have had laryngectomies. Clubs that have joined the Association include Lost Chords, Anamilo, New Voice, and others. At a physician's request, members (who have themselves undergone laryngectomies) visit hospitalized patients to offer emotional support, encouragement, and role models. The Association also extends help to the patient's family and conducts educational and informational programs.

CanSurmount. This support program seeks to improve mutual help and understanding among cancer patients, their families, health professionals, and the community. Its most important function is to arrange (at a physician's request) for visits to the patient and family by a trained CanSurmount volunteer who is also a cancer patient; such visits may take place either at home or in hospital. CanSurmount also promotes programs of continuing education and support for cancer families, health professionals, and community members.

I Can Cope. This program addresses the needs of cancer patients and their families through a series of eight classes. Topics usually covered include: learning about the disease; learning to cope with daily health problems; learning to express feelings; learning to live with limitations; and learning about local resources for cancer families. The lectures, group discussions, and study assignments that make up the course help people with cancer to regain a sense of control over their lives.

CHARTERED DIVISIONS OF THE AMERICAN CANCER SOCIETY

National Headquarters
American Cancer Society, Inc.
777 Third Avenue
New York, New York 10017
   (212) 371-2900

Alabama Division, Inc.
2926 Central Avenue
Birmingham, Alabama 35209
   (205) 879-2242

Alaska Division, Inc.
1343 G Street
Anchorage, Alaska 99501
   (907) 277-8696

Arizona Division, Inc.
634 West Indian School Road
P.O. Box 33187
Phoenix, Arizona 85067
   (602) 264-5861

Arkansas Division, Inc.
5520 West Markham Street
P.O. Box 3822
Little Rock, Arkansas 72203
   (501) 664-3480-1-2

California Division, Inc.
1710 Webster Street
Oakland, California 94612
   (415) 893-7900

Colorado Division, Inc.
1809 East 18th Avenue
P.O. Box 18268
Denver, Colorado 80218
   (303) 321-2464

Connecticut Division, Inc.
Barnes Park South
14 Village Lane
P.O. Box 410
Wallingford, Connecticut 06492
   (203) 265-7161

Delaware Division, Inc.
Academy of Medicine Bldg.
1925 Lovering Avenue
Wilmington, Delaware 19806
(302) 654-6267

District of Columbia Division, Inc.
Universal Building South
1825 Connecticut Avenue, N.W.
Washington, D.C. 20009
(202) 483-2600

Florida Division, Inc.
1001 South MacDill Avenue
Tampa, Florida 33609
(813) 253-0541

Georgia Division, Inc.
1422 W. Peachtree Street, N.W.
Atlanta, Georgia 30309
(404) 892-0026

Hawaii Division, Inc.
Community Services Center Bldg.
200 North Vineyard Boulevard
Honolulu, Hawaii 96817
(808) 531-1662-3-4-5

Idaho Division, Inc.
1609 Abbs Street
P.O. Box 5386
Boise, Idaho 83705
(208) 343-4609

Illinois Division, Inc.
37 South Wabash Avenue
Chicago, Illinois 60603
(312) 372-0472

Indiana Division, Inc.
4755 Kingsway Drive, Suite 100
Indianapolis, Indiana 46205
(317) 257-5326

Iowa Division, Inc.
Highway #18 West
P.O. Box 980
Mason City, Iowa 50401
(515) 423-0712

Kansas Division, Inc.
3003 Van Buren Street
Topeka, Kansas 66611
(913) 267-0131

Kentucky Division, Inc.
Medical Arts Bldg.
1169 Eastern Parkway
Louisville, Kentucky 40217
(502) 459-1867

Louisiana Division, Inc.
Masonic Temple Bldg., Room 810
333 St. Charles Avenue
New Orleans, Louisiana 70130
(504) 523-2029

Maine Division, Inc.
Federal and Green Streets
Brunswick, Maine 04011
(207) 729-3339

Maryland Division, Inc.
200 East Joppa Road
Towson, Maryland 21204
(301) 828-8890

Massachusetts Division, Inc.
247 Commonwealth Avenue
Boston, Massachusetts 02116
(617) 267-2650

Michigan Division, Inc.
1205 East Saginaw Street
Lansing, Michigan 48906
(517) 371-2920

Minnesota Division, Inc.
2750 Park Avenue
Minneapolis, Minnesota 55407
(612) 871-2111

Mississippi Division, Inc.
345 North Mart Plaza
Jackson, Mississippi 39206
(601) 362-8874

Missouri Division, Inc.
715 Jefferson Street
P.O. Box 1066
Jefferson City, Missouri 65101
(314) 636-3195

Montana Division, Inc.
2820 First Avenue South
Billings, Montana 59101
(406) 252-7111

Nebraska Division, Inc.
Overland Wolfe Centre
6910 Pacific Street, Suite 210
Omaha, Nebraska 68106
(402) 551-2422

Nevada Division, Inc.
4100 Boulder Highway
Suite A
Las Vegas, Nevada 89121
(702) 454-4242

New Hampshire Division, Inc.
686 Mast Road
Manchester, New Hampshire 03102
(603) 669-3270

New Jersey Division, Inc.
CN2201
North Brunswick, New Jersey 08902
(201) 297-8000

New Mexico Division, Inc.
5800 Lomas Blvd., N.E.
Albuquerque, New Mexico 87110
(505) 262-1727

New York State Division, Inc.
6725 Lyons Street
P.O. Box 7
East Syracuse, New York 13057
(315) 437-7025

   Long Island Division, Inc.
   535 Broad Hollow Road
   (Route 110)
   Melville, New York 11747
   (516) 420-1111

New York City Division, Inc.
19 West 56th Street
New York, New York 10019
(212) 586-8700

Queens Division, Inc.
111-15 Queens Boulevard
Forest Hills, New York 11375
(212) 263-2224

Westchester Division, Inc.
246 North Central Avenue
Hartsdale, New York 10530
(914) 949-4800

North Carolina Division, Inc.
222 North Person Street
P.O. Box 27624
Raleigh, North Carolina 27611
(919) 834-8463

North Dakota Division, Inc.
Hotel Graver Annex Bldg.
115 Roberts Street
P.O. Box 426
Fargo, North Dakota 58102
(701) 232-1385

Ohio Division, Inc.
453 Lincoln Bldg.
1367 East Sixth Street
Cleveland, Ohio 44114
(216) 771-6700

Oklahoma Division, Inc.
1312 N.W. 24th Street
Oklahoma City, Oklahoma 73106
(405) 525-3515

Oregon Division, Inc.
910 N.E. Union Avenue
Portland, Oregon 97232
(503) 231-5100

Pennsylvania Division, Inc.
Route 422 & Sipe Avenue
P.O. Box 416
Hershey, Pennsylvania 17033
(717) 533-6144

Philadelphia Division, Inc.
21 South 12th Street
Philadelphia, Pennsylvania 19107
(215) 665-2900

Puerto Rico Division, Inc.
(Avenue Domenech 273 Hato Rey,
P.R.)
GPO Box 6004
San Juan, Puerto Rico 00936
(809) 764-2295

Rhode Island Division, Inc.
345 Blackstone Blvd.
Providence, Rhode Island 02906
(401) 831-6970

South Carolina Division, Inc.
2442 Devine Street
Columbia, South Carolina 29205
(803) 256-0245

South Dakota Division, Inc.
1025 North Minnesota Avenue
Hillcrest Plaza
Sioux Falls, South Dakota 57104
(605) 336-0897

Tennessee Division, Inc.
2519 White Avenue
Nashville, Tennessee 37204
(615) 383-1710

Texas Division, Inc.
3834 Spicewood Springs Road
P.O. Box 9863
Austin, Texas 78766
(512) 345-4560

Utah Division, Inc.
610 East South Temple
Salt Lake City, Utah 84102
(801) 322-0431

Vermont Division, Inc.
13 Loomis Street, Drawer C
Montpelier, Vermont 05602
(802) 223-2348

Virginia Division, Inc.
3218 West Cary Street
P.O. Box 7288
Richmond, Virginia 23221
(804) 359-0208

Washington Division, Inc.
2120 First Avenue North
Seattle, Washington 98109
(206) 283-1152

West Virginia Division, Inc.
Suite 100
240 Capital Street
Charleston, West Virginia 25301
(304) 344-3611

Wisconsin Division, Inc.
615 North Sherman Avenue
P.O. Box 8370
Madison, Wisconsin 53708
(608) 249-0487

Milwaukee Division, Inc.
6401 West Capitol Drive
Milwaukee, Wisconsin 53216
(414) 461-1100

Wyoming Division, Inc.
Indian Hills Center
506 Shoshoni
Cheyenne, Wyoming 82001
(307) 638-3331

PUBLICATIONS OF THE AMERICAN CANCER SOCIETY
(PARTIAL LISTING)

Cancer Word Book
Facts on Cancer*
Cancer Facts and Figures
The Hopeful Side of Cancer
Guidelines Concerning Cancer Related
    Check-ups*
Answering the Most Often Asked
    Questions About Cigarette Smoking
    and Lung Cancer
The Beleaguered Lung
A Program of Action Against Cigarette
    Smoking
The Decision Is Yours
When a Woman Smokes
Danger: Cigarettes
Your Health Is Your Business
How to Examine Your Breasts
Facts on Cancer Treatment
What is Chemotherapy?

*Also Available in Spanish

Another Spring: The Diary of a
    Radiation Patient
Cancer Quackery: Laetrile
Facts on . . . Series:
    Bladder Cancer*
    Breast Cancer*
    Cancer of the Larynx*
    Childhood Cancer*
    Colorectal Cancer*
    Hodgkins Disease*
    Leukemia*
    Lung Cancer*
    Oral Cancer*
    Prostate Cancer*
    Skin Cancer*
    Stomach & Esophageal Cancer*
    Testicular Cancer*
    Thyroid Cancer*
    Uterine Cancer*
Curriculum Aids for
    Elementary/Secondary Education

Other Support and Service Organizations

The following national organizations offer information, assistance, and emotional support to cancer patients and their families. In each case, services are provided by local chapters which may be located in a local telephone directory or through the respective national office.

Leukemia Society of America, Inc.

800 Second Avenue
New York, New York 10017
    (212) 573-8484

Local chapters of the Society offer patients with leukemia and related disorders a range of services including financial assistance, transportation, and consultations that may lead to referrals to other sources of local support.

Make Today Count
P.O. Box 303
Burlington, Iowa 52601
    (319) 753-6112 or (319) 754-8977
More than 200 chapters of this organization have been founded by cancer patients, people with other life-threatening diseases, their families, health care professionals, and interested members of the local community. Chapters are organized informally and typically hold one or two meetings each month. The organization's goals are to provide emotional self-helf and to help each patient and family to live each day as fully and as completely as possible.

United Cancer Council, Inc.
1803 North Meridian Street
Indianapolis, Indiana 46202
    (317) 923-6490
This federation of voluntary cancer agencies is funded through the United Way of Giving in most communities where they are located. Member agencies provide services that include nursing, homemaking and housekeeping, medications and prostheses, and rehabilitation.

United Ostomy Association, Inc.
2001 West Beverly Boulevard
Los Angeles, California 90057
    (213) 413-5510
Members of the more than 500 chapters nationwide include persons who have had colostomy, ileostomy, or urostomy surgery, although not all members are cancer patients. The Association offers mutual aid, emotional support, and education to persons with common problems.

Guidelines suggested by the American Cancer Society for the early detection of cancer in people without symptoms

Age 20–40	Age 40 & Over

Cancer-related checkup every 3 years
Should include the procedures listed below plus health counseling (such as tips on quitting cigarettes) and examinations for cancers of the thyroid, testes, prostate, mouth, ovaries, skin and lymph nodes. Some people are at higher risk for certain cancers and may need to have tests more frequently.

Cancer-related checkup every year
Should include the procedures listed below plus health counseling (such as tips on quitting cigarettes) and examinations for cancers of the thyroid, testes, prostate, mouth, ovaries, skin and lymph nodes. Some people are at higher risk for certain cancers and may need to have tests more frequently.

Breast
- Exam by doctor every 3 years
- Self-exam every month
- One baseline breast X-ray between ages 35–40

    Higher Risk for Breast Cancer: Personal or family history of breast cancer, never had children, first child after 30

Breast
- Exam by doctor every year
- Self-exam every month
- Breast X-ray every year after 50 (betweens ages 40–50, ask your doctor)

    Higher Risk for Breast Cancer: Personal or family history of breast cancer, never had children, first child after 30

Uterus
- Pelvic exam every 3 years

Cervix
- Pap test—after 2 initial negative tests 1 year apart—*at least* every 3 years, includes women under 20 if sexually active

    Higher Risk for Cervical Cancer: Early age at first intercourse, multiple sex partners

Uterus
- Pelvic exam every year

Cervix
- Pap test—after 2 initial negative tests 1 year apart—*at least* every 3 years

    Higher Risk for Cervical Cancer: Early age at first intercourse, multiple sex partners

Endometrium
- Endometrial tissue sample at menopause if at risk

    Higher Risk for Endometrial Cancer: Infertility, obesity, failure of ovulation, abnormal uterine bleeding, estrogen therapy

---

Remember, these guidelines are not rules and only apply to people without symptoms. If you have any of the 7 Warning Signals see your doctor or go to your clinic without delay.

Colon & rectum
- Digital rectal exam every year
- Guaiac slide test every year after 50
- Proto exam—after 2 initial negative tests 1 year apart—every 3 to 5 years after 50

    Higher Risk for Colorectal Cancer: Personal or family history of colon or rectal cancer, personal or family history of polyps in the colon or rectum, ulcerative colitis

A pamphlet entitled *Guidelines Concerning Cancer Related Check-ups* is available from the American Cancer Society.

Index